REFLEXOLOGY

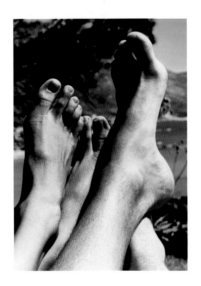

an introduction to
REFLEXOLOGY

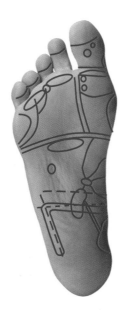

Joëlle Peeters

p

This is a Parragon book
This edition published in 2005

Parragon
Queen Street House
4 Queen Street
Bath BA1 1HE, UK

Copyright © Parragon 2002

This book was created by
THE BRIDGEWATER BOOK COMPANY

Photography Ian Parsons

A CIP catalogue record for this book is available from the British Library

ISBN 1-40544-621-8

Printed in Indonesia

Contents

What Is **Reflexology?**	6
How Does **Reflexology** Work?	8
Anatomy	12
Elements	20
Introduction to **Reflex Maps**	22
The Anatomy of the **Foot**	24
The **Head**	26
The **Thoracic** and **Upper Abdominal** Area	28
The **Lower Abdominal** Area	30
The **Pelvic** Area	32
The **Reproductive** Area	33
The **Spine**	34
The **Outer Foot**	36
The **Top** of the **Foot**	37
Symptoms and **Case Histories**	38
Basic **Techniques**	40
Massage Techniques	42
Relaxing the **Foot**	44

The **Main Treatment** 46

Reactions Following a Treatment 56

Diseases and their
Associated Reflex Areas 58

Respiratory Problems 60

Heart, Blood and
Circulatory Problems 62

Digestive Problems 64

Reproductive Problems 68

Aches and **Pains** 70

Ears, Eyes, Mouth and **Throat** 72

Skin and **Hair** Problems 74

Allergies 76

Nervous Disorders 78

Treating Yourself 80

Reflex Maps of the Hands 82

The **Head** 84

The **Thoracic** and **Upper**
Abdominal Area 86

The **Lower Abdominal** and
Pelvic Areas 88

The **Reproductive Reflexes** 90

The **Limb Reflexes** 92

Lymphatics and **Breast Area** 93

Glossary 94

Useful Addresses 95

Index 96

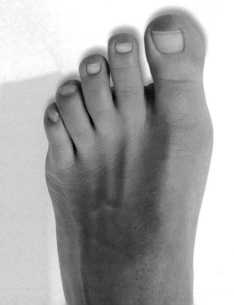
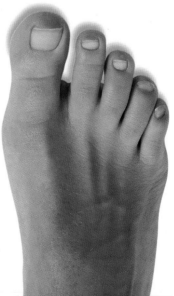

What Is **Reflexology?**

Reflexology functions in two ways: as a diagnostic tool, and as a method of treatment. A reflexology treatment can be used for the correction and prevention of ill health.

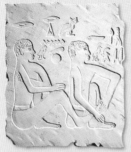

Drawings from the tomb of Ankm'ahor, a powerful physician in Ancient Egypt.

It is known that different reflex points found in the feet and hands correspond to areas in the body. By using the thumb and fingers in a particular way to massage the relevant reflex points, pain and other symptoms in the corresponding area of the body can be alleviated. This knowledge probably originated in China, where the Chinese used pressure points on the feet as a form of treatment as long as 5,000 years ago.

The earliest pictorial evidence of reflexology was discovered in the tomb of a physician named Ankm'ahor, at Saqqara in Egypt, dating from around 2500 to 2330BCE. The tomb drawings show practitioners massaging their patients' hands and feet, with inscription reading 'do not hurt me', and 'I shall act so you shall praise me'. Evidence has shown that, in more recent times, Native American folk medicine also used a form of foot massage as a healing aid.

Knowledge of the reflex points on the feet may have been passed to indigenous Americans by the Incas.

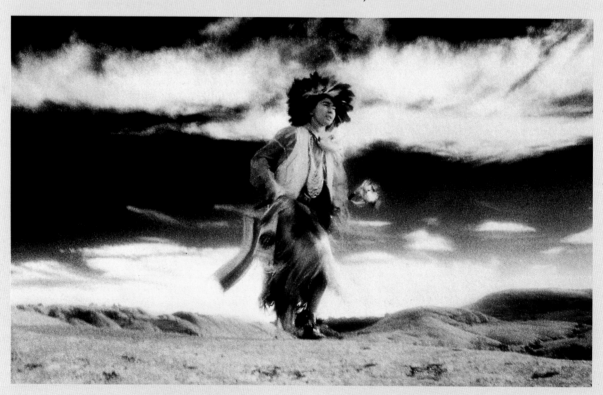

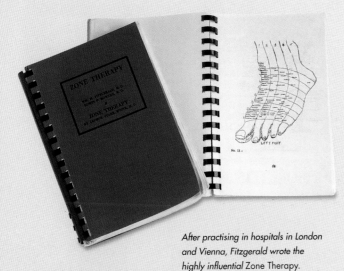

After practising in hospitals in London and Vienna, Fitzgerald wrote the highly influential Zone Therapy.

In 1917 Dr William H Fitzgerald, an ear, nose and throat consultant in America, published the book *Zone Therapy, or Relieving pain at home.* He divided the body into ten longitudinal zones (or energy channels) – hence the term 'zone therapy'.

Dr Fitzgerald observed that by using, for example, elastic bands or metal combs to apply pressure to fingers or toes, he could bring about an anaesthetizing effect and normalization to all parts of the zone treated.

Eunice Ingham trained as a remedial therapist, and so had a paramedical background. She is known as 'the mother of reflexology' for her work on mapping each reflex and point of contact on the hands and feet to the various organs and glands of the body. She also developed the 'Ingham Compression Method of Reflexology'. Her two books, *Stories the Feet can Tell* and *Stories the Feet Have Told,* are now standard textbooks for the reflexology student. She had her own successful practice, lectured, and trained many practitioners in America.

Mrs Doreen E Bayly, a British nurse, discovered reflexology for herself when she went to visit her sister, a healer in America. While there, she met Eunice Ingham and studied with her, returning to Britain in the early 1960s. Doreen Bayly managed, despite encountering some opposition at first, to make reflexology known in Britain and Europe. She also built up a successful practice, and founded the Bayly School of Reflexology.

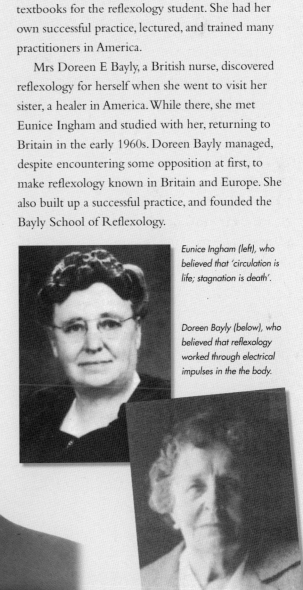

Eunice Ingham (left), who believed that 'circulation is life; stagnation is death'.

Doreen Bayly (below), who believed that reflexology worked through electrical impulses in the the body.

How Does
Reflexology Work?

In common with many holistic therapies, reflexology works on the principle that energy balance will lead to greater vitality.

The body has ten longitudinal zones, which run from the tip of the fingers and thumbs, up through the brain, and down to the tip of the toes. Five zones are found on either side of the median (or central) line of the body. These zones are like longitudinal sections through the body, extending from front to back and containing the internal organs and glands of that section.

In natural medicine the energy within us is known as the 'life force', or 'vital energy' (in Traditional Chinese Medicine, this same life force is known as *qi*). The longitudinal zones or energy channels used in reflexology are considered to be paths along which someone's vital energy flows. So if an organ is present in one or more zones, the corresponding reflex area will be found within the same zone(s) in the hands or feet. Stress, disease and injury can all lead to congestion along these energy pathways.

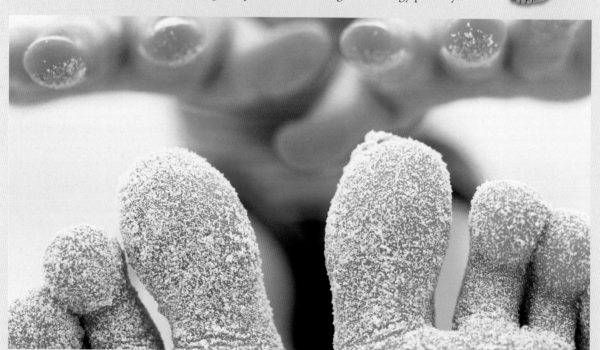

Leonardo da Vinci described the human foot as a masterpiece of engineering and a work of art.

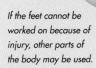

If the feet cannot be worked on because of injury, other parts of the body may be used.

Every part of the foot or hand contains reflex areas which correspond to a part of the body. The feet (soles, tops and sides) are more commonly used in reflexology than other parts of the body because their reflexes are more responsive.

LONGITUDINAL ZONES

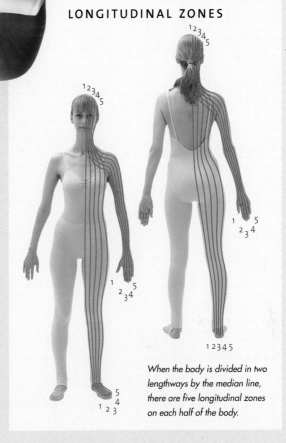

When the body is divided in two lengthways by the median line, there are five longitudinal zones on each half of the body.

FOOT AND HAND ZONES

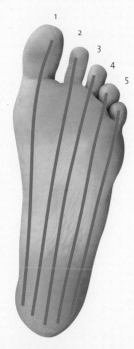

Although reflexology is an ancient art, Dr William H Fitzgerald was the first person to describe how the longitudinal zones in the body correspond to the zones of the feet and hands.

Each finger and each toe falls into one of the five zones to be found on that side of the body, and points in that zone can be used to treat the related areas.

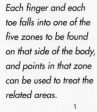

Reflexology, being a holistic therapy, uses the principle of the whole being present in each part. No one body part works in isolation; every part works together for the benefit of all. Thus the build-up of toxins in one part of the body eventually leads to different parts having to work harder to compensate for the imbalance in body energies. By stimulating the various reflexes on the feet and hands, it is possible to clear away the congestion of toxic deposits that inhibit the flow of the vital force through our bodies, thereby bringing about a state of equilibrium or balance (homeostasis) within the body. This improves our health and vitality.

Exactly how massaging a reflex in the foot or hand can produce a measurable effect on another part of the body within that zone is not fully understood. It is, however, accepted that a reflexology treatment has a beneficial effect on the blood circulation and the nervous system.

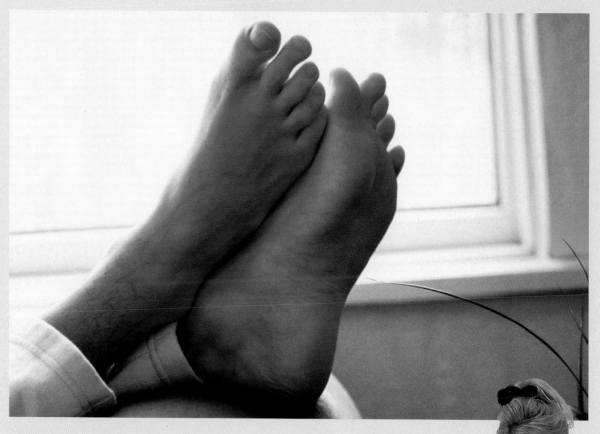

THE EFFECT OF REFLEXOLOGY
ON THE CIRCULATION SYSTEM

Exposed and hard-working, the feet themselves are particularly vulnerable to circulatory disorders.

The truth of Eunice Ingham's famous saying 'Circulation is life; stagnation is death' can be shown by the effect of cutting off the blood supply to even the smallest part of the body. Soon a variety of aches and pains occur, and the colour starts changing; if the blockage continues, the affected part eventually will die. We all know that our hands and feet will respond to cold conditions by starting to ache; this is because cold has the effect of reducing the bloody supply. Organs and glands that do not receive a sufficiently rich supply of blood malfunction and lose their balancing qualities. The body then slowly stops being a harmonious unit.

Tension has the effect of restricting blood flow, causing high or low blood pressure. High blood pressure can cause thickening of the blood vessel walls. Materials build up, coating the inside of the arteries, and this is called hardening of the arteries or arteriosclerosis. When the blood flow is reduced because of the build-up in the artery, the kidney releases the hormone renin, which further increases blood pressure. Reflexology causes the body to become more relaxed. This facilitates a sufficiently rich supply of blood to the organs and glands, and so they start functioning in a more harmonious state.

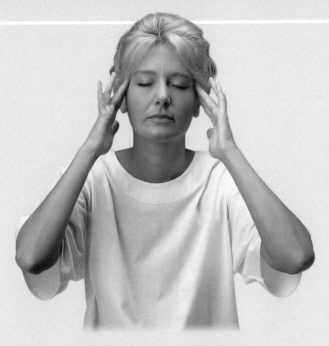

Tension headache is a common condition that causes misery for many people; the answer could lie in a rebalancing of your bodily energies.

THE EFFECT OF REFLEXOLOGY ON THE NERVOUS SYSTEM

The nerves, which are cord-like structures, convey impulses from the central nervous system to other parts of the body. By this type of communication they are able to co-ordinate the function of the organs and the various body parts, to enable them to work in equilibrium with one another.

Tension can put pressure on various nerves, causing messages to the organs to be impaired. This often means that the organ will not function as it should. Many of us have had personal experience of this – 'tension' headaches are an example.

Reflexology stimulates thousands of nerve endings, and thereby encourages the opening and clearing of neural pathways. Reflexology also reduces tension, and so aids the nervous system.

In Western cultures it is quite rare for a child to receive reflexology, but other cultures have known for centuries that this therapy can be effective for everyone.

BENEFITS AND CAUTION

A large proportion, approximately 75 per cent, of disorders and diseases are brought about by external influences, like stress and lifestyle factors. People react to these stresses and tensions in various ways. One person may have backaches, another cardiovascular problems, another may become more nervous.

However, anyone who is willing to accept responsibility for their own well-being can benefit from a reflexology treatment. Reflexology does not discriminate – anyone, from babies right up to the elderly, can gain relief from it.

By stimulating the elimination of waste materials from the body, or improving the circulation, it is possible to speed up the healing process, thereby normalizing bodily functions.

Most disorders will benefit from a reflexology treatment; however, it is unsuitable for some (see page 57 for details).

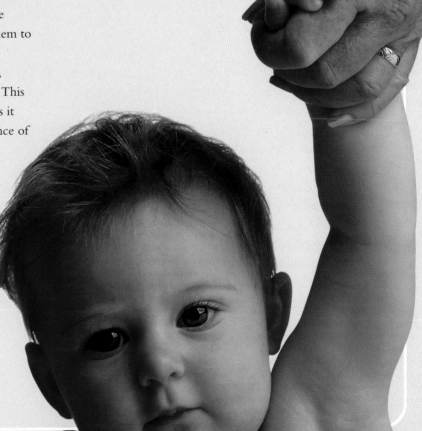

Anatomy

As already discussed, reflexology is a holistic therapy; among other things, this means that all of the following bodily systems need to be taken into account, and they must work harmoniously together to produce a physically and mentally healthy person.

SKELETAL SYSTEM

The bones give the body support and protect the internal glands and organs. They also give the body its shape, and they regulate minerals, particularly calcium, phosphorous, copper and cobalt. Healthy bone marrow is vital, as it manufactures red and white blood as well as platelet cells.

MUSCULAR SYSTEM

Muscles are composed of tissue which can be contracted so that movement can occur. They convert energy from food and respiration into physical movement, usually in response to signals from the brain and the nervous system. They make up 35–45 per cent of the average person's weight.

There are three main types of muscle tissue.
Skeletal This type of muscle tissue is under the mind's conscious control, and it will respond to nervous signals by controlling the movement of the relevant skeletal bone (for example, the biceps pulls on the humerus to elevate the upper arm). There are over 650 skeletal muscles throughout the body.
Smooth This is found in the intestines and the linings of organs, and is not under conscious control.
Cardiac This is a special type of involuntary tissue and is found only in the heart.

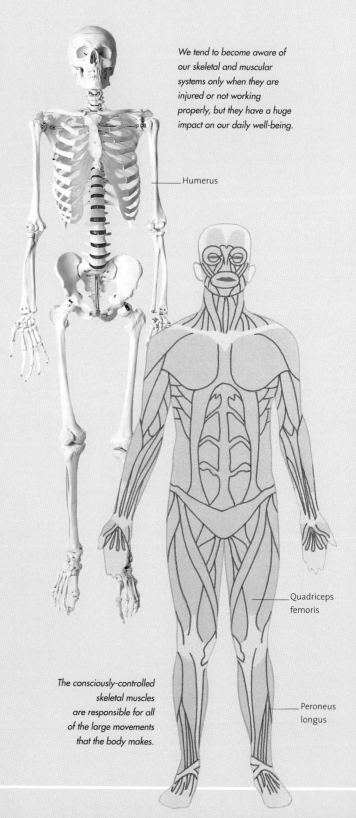

We tend to become aware of our skeletal and muscular systems only when they are injured or not working properly, but they have a huge impact on our daily well-being.

Humerus

Quadriceps femoris

Peroneus longus

The consciously-controlled skeletal muscles are responsible for all of the large movements that the body makes.

NERVOUS SYSTEM

The nervous system is made up of two parts.

The central nervous system This consists of the brain and spinal cord.

The peripheral nervous system This carries information from various parts of the body, through the relevant sensory nerves to the central nervous system. It carries out instructions through the efferent motor nerves (nerve cells which carry impulses away from the central nervous system to related parts of the body). The nerves are made up of thousands of long thin nerve fibres. Like all other organ systems, the nervous system consists of different types of cells.

CIRCULATORY SYSTEM

The heart, an organ about the size of a clenched fist, is situated in the thorax. The heart pumps deoxygenated blood to the lungs, where carbon dioxide and oxygen are exchanged. This happens through the alveolar surface (a thin-walled air-filled sac which is surrounded by blood capillaries) of the lung. Oxygenated blood returns to the heart. This is known as the pulmonary circulation. The systemic circulation carries the oxygenated blood and nutrition to all the other parts of the body, returning with the waste products that have to be filtered and excreted. Carbon dioxide is also returned to the heart by the systemic circulatory system, where, after being pumped through the heart chambers, it enters the pulmonary circulatory system, and so the process starts again.

Although the circulatory system of an adult contains only ten pints of blood, the heart is powerful enough to pump it all around the body.

Brain

Spinal cord

Peripheral nervous system

Sympathetic nervous system

The central nervous system (left) consists of the brain and the spinal cord, and together with the sympathetic and peripheral systems it controls movement in the body.

Deoxygenated blood

Oxygenated blood

The circulatory system (above), containing the heart itself as well as blood circulation network.

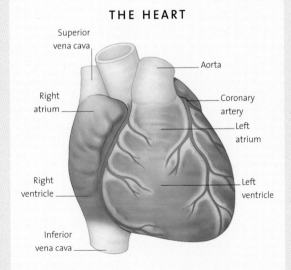

THE HEART

Superior vena cava

Aorta

Right atrium

Coronary artery

Left atrium

Right ventricle

Left ventricle

Inferior vena cava

LYMPHATIC SYSTEM

This is our defence system for protecting the body from bacteria and other organisms. Lymph is transported by the lymphatic system. Lymph nodes are situated at intervals along the lymphatics. The lymph nodes contain a system of narrow channels through which the lymph drains in. Along the walls of these channels, large phagocytes (cells that engulf particles) surround bacteria, other harmful substances and dead cells from the lymph. Large lymph nodes are found in the neck, under the arms, in the breast and in the groin. The large lymphatics unite into two lymphatic ducts, which then drain into the bloodstream. The spleen and the thymus are also part of the lymphatic system. The spleen is a large vascular ductless organ found on the left side of the body behind the stomach. It plays an important part in the immune system, producing lymphocytes (white blood cells), and is involved in the breakdown and recycling of haemoglobin from old blood cells.

RESPIRATORY SYSTEM

The human respiratory system is made up of the nose and mouth, the pharynx and larynx in the throat, and the windpipe or tracheae. The tracheae then divides into two bronchi, which enter the lungs. The bronchi subdivide into smaller bronchioles, and they in turn subdivide into the alveolar ducts of the alveolar sacs, which contain the individual alveoli. The main muscles used in breathing are the intercostal muscles (these run in between the ribs and the diaphragm).

Respiration in humans is the process by which oxygen is converted during metabolism to produce carbon dioxide. This gaseous exchange occurs through the alveoli in the lungs.

The respiratory system (right). Reflexology treatments can be used to target the respiratory functions, encouraging clear breathing as well as clearing congestion.

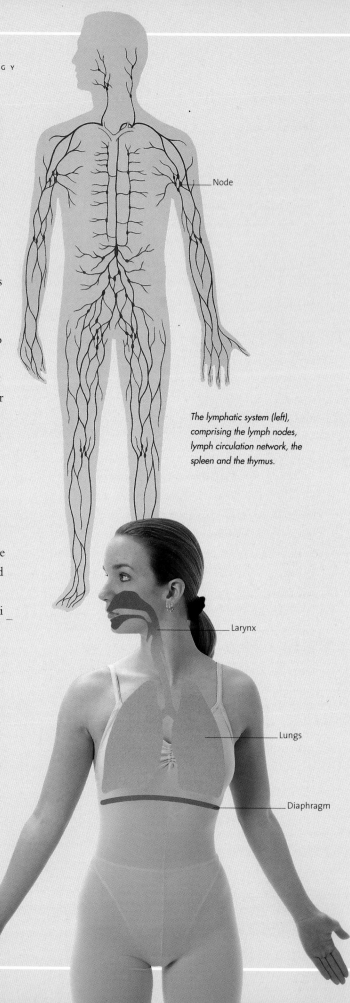

Node

The lymphatic system (left), comprising the lymph nodes, lymph circulation network, the spleen and the thymus.

Larynx

Lungs

Diaphragm

URINARY SYSTEM

The urinary system consists of the two kidneys, situated on either side of the spine. They filter the blood, and regulate the composition and volume of body fluids by eliminating what cannot be reused, for example salts, waste products and excess water. Renal arteries and veins bring a rich blood supply to and from the kidneys. The kidneys are connected to the bladder by the ureter tubes. Urine continuously drains out of the kidneys into the ureters and into the bladder. This constant flow of urine into the bladder causes it to swell. The bladder wall contains sensory nerve endings which send messages to the brain, alerting the person when the bladder needs to be emptied. By relaxing the sphincter muscle around the urethra, urination can then occur.

ENDOCRINE SYSTEM

The endocrine system consists of ductless glands which produce and secrete hormones directly into the bloodstream. These hormones are carried in the blood until they affect those organs that are sensitive to them. Both the nervous system and the endocrine system co-ordinate the body's activities, but they do this in different ways.

The endocrine glands include the pituitary gland, which is found in the brain. The activity of the pituitary is regulated by the hypothalamus, which is found just above the pituitary. The pituitary gland controls the function of the thyroid, adrenals and the reproductive glands (the ovaries and testes).

The parathyroid glands, the pancreas, the placenta and gastrointestinal mucosa are also part of the endocrine system.

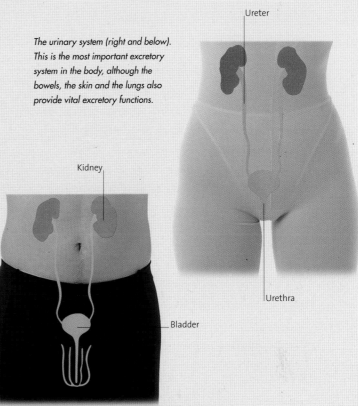

The urinary system (right and below). This is the most important excretory system in the body, although the bowels, the skin and the lungs also provide vital excretory functions.

Ureter

Kidney

Urethra

Bladder

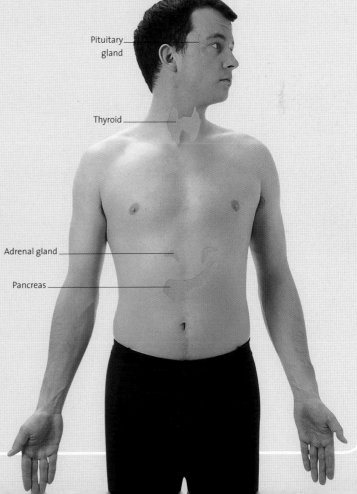

Pituitary gland

Thyroid

Adrenal gland

Pancreas

The endocrine system (right). The hormones that are produced and circulated by the endocrine system have important effects on growth, reproduction and states of emotion.

REPRODUCTIVE SYSTEM

Most of the male reproductive anatomy is external. The two testes hang in scrotal sacs. Two long convoluted tubes called the epididymis, one on each side, are attached to the testes. These allow the sperm which have been produced in the testes to ripen. The epididymis then opens into the vas deferens, another two long tubes – one on each side of the body – which are joined to the seminal vesicles. The seminal vesicles act as a storage place for mature sperm before they are released through the centre of the prostate gland and the urethra.

The female reproductive organs consist of the ovaries, Fallopian tubes, the uterus and the breasts.

The testes and ovaries produce reproductive cells that are called spermatozoa and ova. They also produce hormones that influence body development and behaviour.

DIGESTIVE SYSTEM

Digestion starts in the mouth. Food is chewed and mixed with saliva, which contains enzymes that make a start on the process of breaking larger molecules down into smaller ones which are more easily absorbed. The saliva also lubricates the food, making it softer and easier to swallow.

The ingested food then enters the oesophagus and travels to the stomach. Here it is churned and mixed together with the stomach acids that change the food substances into a state that is more easily absorbed. The mixture then enters the small intestine and the large intestine, where further breakdown and absorption take place. The unabsorbed residue is expelled through the rectum and anus.

The liver, gall bladder and pancreas are also important in the digestion process.

The digestive system (right). This is responsible for the ingestion, storage and excretion of food and waste products, and is easily affected by stress.

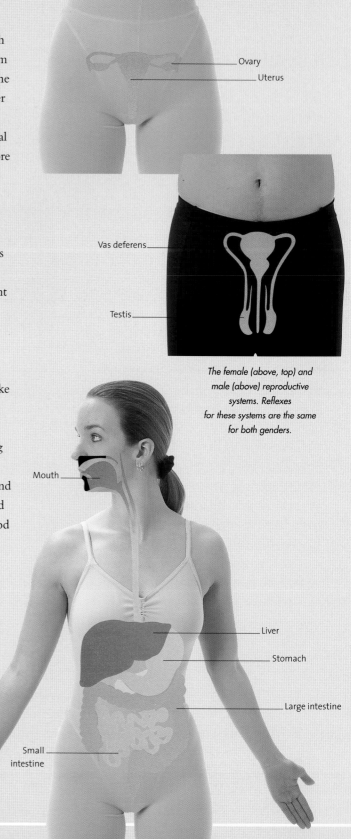

Ovary
Uterus
Vas deferens
Testis

The female (above, top) and male (above) reproductive systems. Reflexes for these systems are the same for both genders.

Mouth
Liver
Stomach
Large intestine
Small intestine

SENSORY SYSTEM

The sense organs allow the body to be aware of its environment by working in the following way. When a sensory cell is stimulated, electrical impulses are sent along nerve pathways to the brain. Once the signals arrive at the appropriate part of the brain they are interpreted as sight, sound, pain and so on. The following organs are part of the sensory system.

The skin This is a waterproof protective layer around the body which protects us from shock and infection. It regulates our body temperature and is sensitive to touch, temperature, pressure and pain. The skin also has an important excretory function.

The eyes These complex organs allow us to see by the use of the cornea (which aids focusing), a lens, an adjustable iris with the pupil at its centre, and the retina, which contains millions of light-sensitive cells. The visual information is then carried to the brain by nerves. The eyes, which are circular in shape, are housed in the skull in depressions called orbits. Each eye is attached to the wall of the orbit by six muscles, which can also move the eyeball.

The ears The ear is made up of three parts. The outer ear picks up sound and sends it to the middle ear, which contains the ear-drum and three small bones. These magnify the sound before sending it to the inner ear, which houses the cochlea, a snail-shell-like structure containing microscopic nerve cells, each one of which is sensitive to a certain vibration. The vibrations produce an electric current which is carried by the auditory nerve to the brain, where it is decoded into what we know as 'sound' or 'noise'.

The inner ear is also responsible for balance. The three semi-circular canals are filled with a fluid which sends messages to the brain by means of tiny hairs and nerves in the ear, allowing the person to maintain their equilibrium.

The sensory system (right) takes inputs from the eyes, nose, mouth, ears and skin (among others) and converts them into information that our brains can work with.

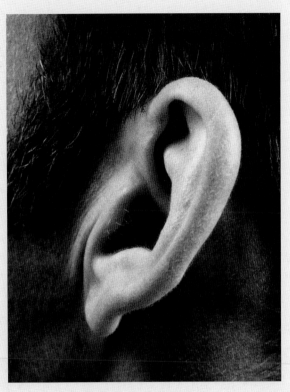

The ear is not only the organ of hearing; it also has an important part to play in maintaining the body's equilibrium.

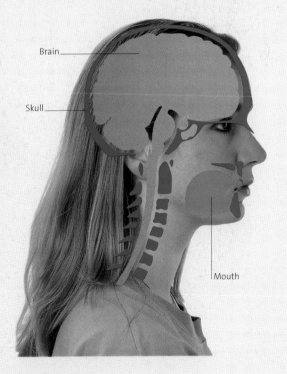

Brain

Skull

Mouth

The nose The nose has numerous functions. Its primary use is in breathing, during which it filters out particles from the air through the nasal hairs and mucous before the air enters the lungs.

The nose has the capacity to recognize different smells. The olfactory organs, which are sensitive to smell, are found in the upper regions of the nasal cavity. When chemical molecules stimulate these organs, nerve endings will send the messages to the olfactory part of the brain, where they are decoded.

The sense of smell is easily fatigued, so that after a few minutes' exposure to a new smell, the smell is no longer perceived. It should be noted that the senses of smell and taste are closely linked. This is why, when the nasal cavity is congested – such as when one has a cold – the sense of taste is also affected. Smokers also find that their senses of smell and taste are adversely affected.

The tongue The tongue contains various muscles that run in different directions, which allows it to be a highly mobile organ. This is important in the chewing process, as well as in swallowing and speech. The tongue is also sensitive to temperature, touch and, of course, taste. Taste buds are located on the surface of the tongue among the 9,000 or so tiny projections which are called papillae.

All flavours are made up of a mixture of the four basic tastes: sweet and salty (which can be detected by taste buds at the front of the tongue); sour (which can be found on the side of the tongue about half-way up); and bitter (which can be detected at the back of the tongue).

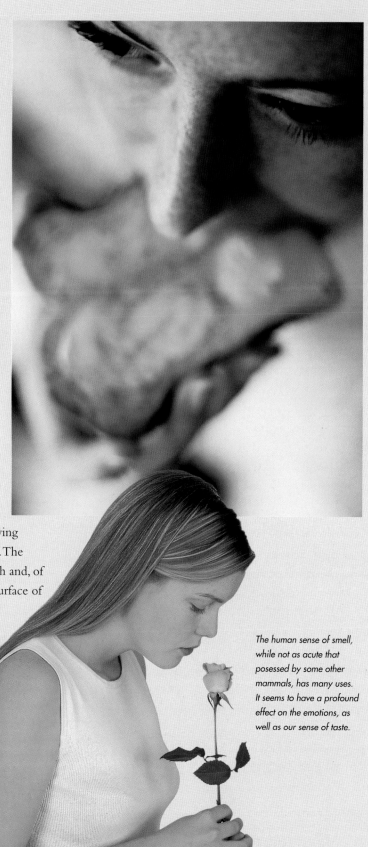

The human sense of smell, while not as acute that posessed by some other mammals, has many uses. It seems to have a profound effect on the emotions, as well as our sense of taste.

MERIDIANS

Traditional Chinese Medicine classifies 1,000 or so acupuncture points into 12 main groups. An imaginary line joins all the acupuncture points belonging to any one of these groups. These lines are what we refer to as 'meridians'. The meridians are energy pathways, along which flows the vital life force which is sometimes called qi. As with the reflexology zones that we have discussed previously, they are duplicated on each side of the body, with two central meridians (known as the 'governing' and 'conception' meridians) running down the front and back of the body along its central or median line.

When there is a build-up of toxins along a certain meridian, this causes a congestion of the energy. This congestion will affect the organ associated with that meridian (for example, the lung in the lung meridian) which will suffer a lack of energy. By stimulating one or more acupuncture points on the meridian using reflexology techniques, the congestion is eased, returning the organ to a harmonious state.

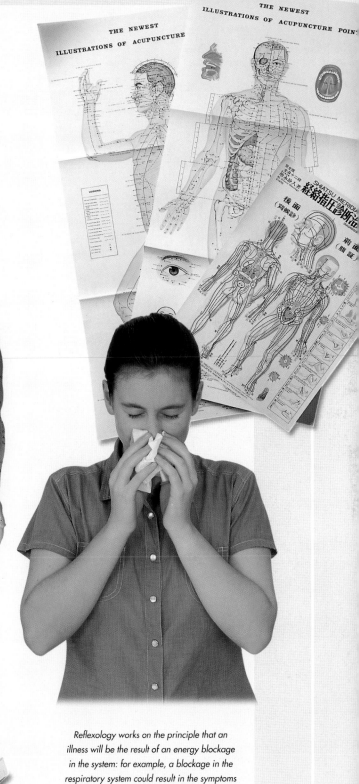

Meridians and acupuncture points on the body, shown by a model and charts (right and top right). Knowledge of the meridians has been passed down to us through ancient Chinese techniques.

Reflexology works on the principle that an illness will be the result of an energy blockage in the system: for example, a blockage in the respiratory system could result in the symptoms of the common cold.

Elements

Everything on the Earth can be classified into one or more of the five elements. These are wood, fire, earth, metal and water. In Traditional Chinese Medicine, these five elements form two cycles – the creative cycle and the destructive cycle.

THE CREATIVE CYCLE

Wood will burn to create fire, which when it has finished burning produces ashes (earth). Earth contains metals, which when heated will become molten, like water – which is necessary for the growth of plants and wood.

The creative element cycle (below). The ancient Chinese theory of the elements is related to the Daoist philosophical beliefs that dominate traditional Chinese culture.

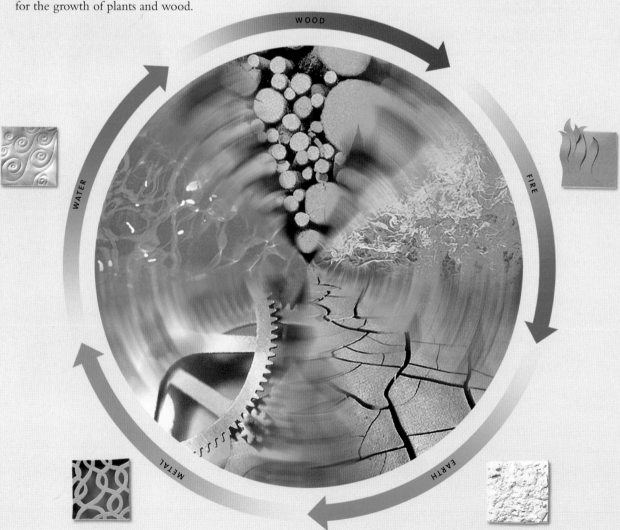

WOOD

FIRE

EARTH

METAL

WATER

THE DESTRUCTIVE CYCLE

Wood destroys earth – the roots of plants and trees can break up the soil. Earth destroys water – its earthen banks contain a pond. Water destroys fire. Fire destroys metal – a metal object will eventually melt when it is placed in the fire. Metal destroys wood – a metal saw or axe can cut a tree down.

In Traditional Chinese Medicine, the law of the five elements is as follows.

• Wood is associated with the liver and the gall bladder.

• Fire is associated with the heart, pericardium, triple burner and small intestine.

• Earth is associated with the spleen and stomach.

• Metal is associated with the lung and large intestine.

• Water is associated with the kidneys and bladder.

By using the theory of the five elements one can understand that, for example, when the liver (wood) is tonified, the heart (fire) will also be tonified, while the stomach and spleen (earth) will be sedated. Looking at another example, if the kidneys (water) are sedated, the liver (wood) will also be sedated, and the heart (fire) will be tonified.

This relationship between the five elements and their associated organs helps the practitioner to understand unexpected results when carrying out a reflexology treatment.

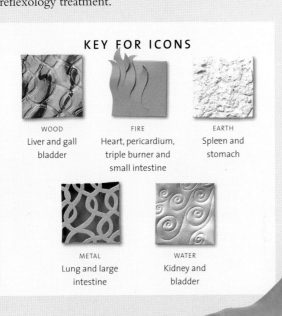

KEY FOR ICONS

WOOD
Liver and gall bladder

FIRE
Heart, pericardium, triple burner and small intestine

EARTH
Spleen and stomach

METAL
Lung and large intestine

WATER
Kidney and bladder

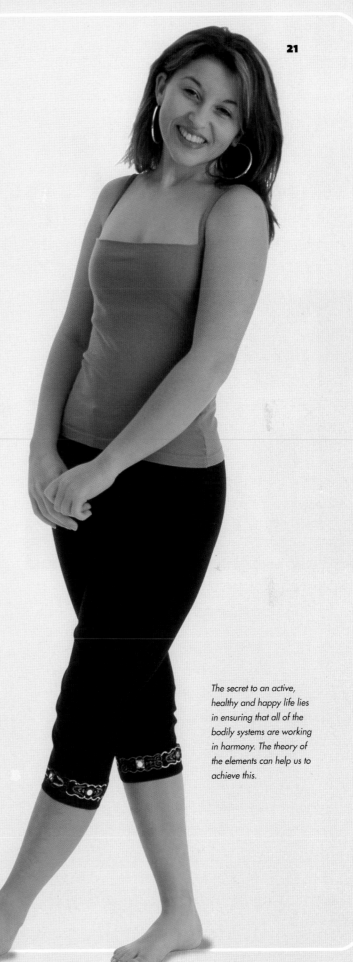

The secret to an active, healthy and happy life lies in ensuring that all of the bodily systems are working in harmony. The theory of the elements can help us to achieve this.

Introduction to
Reflex Maps

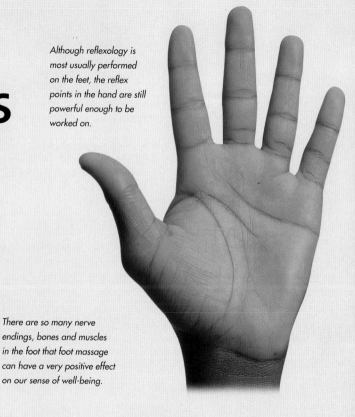

Although reflexology is most usually performed on the feet, the reflex points in the hand are still powerful enough to be worked on.

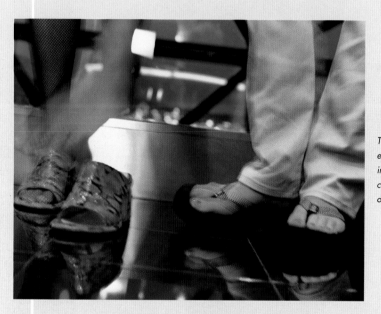

There are so many nerve endings, bones and muscles in the foot that foot massage can have a very positive effect on our sense of well-being.

REFLEX MAPS OF THE FOOT AND
THEIR RELATIONSHIP TO THE BODY PARTS

One of the most important parts of reflexology is a thorough understanding of the feet in relation to the body. The feet are like a small map of the whole body. All the organs, glands and various body parts are imaged on the feet in almost the same arrangement as in the body. Reflex areas are found on the soles, sides and tops of the feet. The hands also contain reflex areas on their palms, sides and backs.

The body is therefore divided into two halves. The right foot represents the right side of the body while the medial (inside) of the foot represents the right half of the spine. The left foot represents the left side of the body, with the medial representing the left half of the spine.

Perhaps it should be pointed out that the right side of the brain is located in the right foot and the left side in the left foot. The zones do not cross in the brain as the nervous system does.

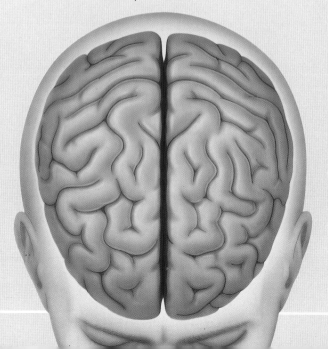

The left-hand side of our brain controls the right-hand side of our body and vice versa, but this is not the case in reflexology.

ALL-ROUND WELL-BEING

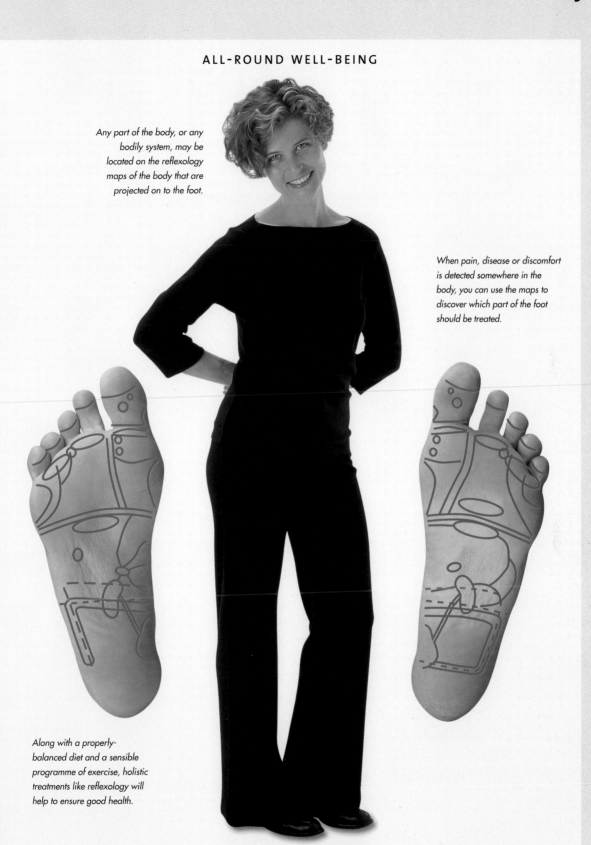

Any part of the body, or any bodily system, may be located on the reflexology maps of the body that are projected on to the foot.

When pain, disease or discomfort is detected somewhere in the body, you can use the maps to discover which part of the foot should be treated.

Along with a properly-balanced diet and a sensible programme of exercise, holistic treatments like reflexology will help to ensure good health.

The Anatomy of the **Foot**

The feet bear the whole of the body weight. The heel, the base of the big toe and the base of the little toe form a kind of three-dimensional arch which supports the body weight. The feet also act as a springboard for walking and running.

The many muscles, the numerous ligaments and the bones that make up the foot create systems of fulcrums and levers, which makes the feet strong and flexible.

• Each foot is made up of 26 bones.

• Each toe is made up of three bones (except the big toe, which has only two). These bones are called the phalanges.

• Below the phalanges are the five metatarsals. These link each toe to the other bones of the foot.

• The cuboid bone is found under the little and fourth toe metatarsals.

• The side protrusion on the cuboid bone is called the cuboid notch. The three smaller cuneiforms are found under the big toe, the second and third toes. The navicular is positioned below the cuneiforms.

• The calcaneum (heel bone) and the talus are found in the heel region of the foot.

• The cuboid, cuneiforms, navicular, calcaneum and the talus are grouped together and are known as the tarsal bones.

• Each foot is divided into five longitudinal zones, each zone containing one toe. The foot is then further divided into eight sections.

• The head and neck is represented by the toes. The right foot represents the right side of the head with its associated organs, and the left foot the left side of the head with its various organs.

• The thoracic and upper abdominal area (from the shoulders to the diaphragm, most of the stomach and part of the kidneys) is represented by the ball of the foot, or more precisely the area between the base of the phalanges to the base of the metatarsal bones. The line at the base of the metatarsal bones is often referred to as the waistline, and can be more easily located by running a horizontal line across the foot from the cuboid notch.

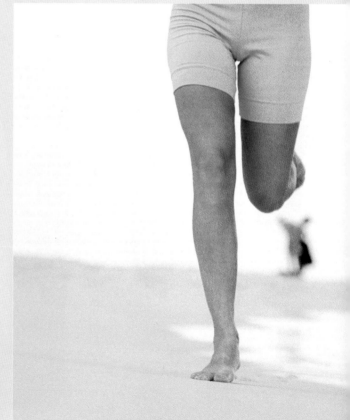

The foot supports an enormous amount of weight for its size. When we evolved into two-legged creatures, our feet suddenly had to do twice as much work as before.

• The lower abdominal area (from the lower part of the stomach and kidneys to the pelvis) is represented on the foot by the area between the waistline and the pelvic line. This is located by connecting the inner and outer ankle-bone protrusions (malleoli), which run under the foot. Thus, the reflexes of the abdomen and pelvis are found over the tarsal bones and around the ankle-bones.

• The pelvic area is represented by the heel, running from the pelvic line to the rear of the heel.

• The reproductive area is represented by different parts of the ankle.

• The spine is represented by the instep. The curve of a person's spine will closely resemble the natural sweep of their instep.

• The arms and legs are represented by the outer edges of the foot.

• The reflexes for the breasts and the lymphatic system are on the top of the foot.

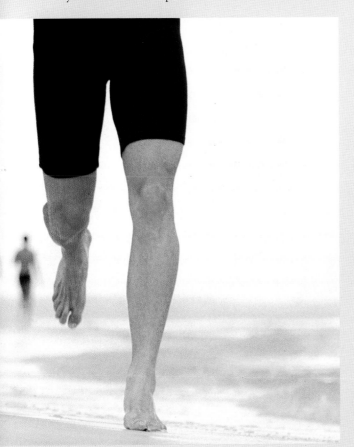

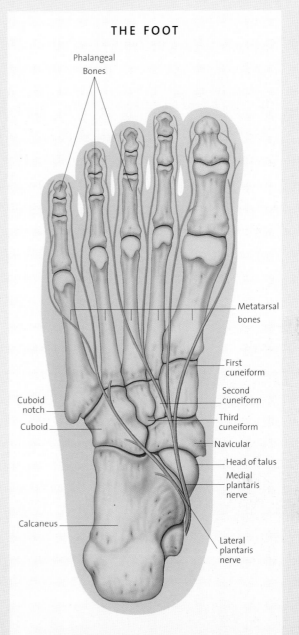

THE FOOT

Phalangeal Bones

Metatarsal bones

First cuneiform

Second cuneiform

Cuboid notch

Third cuneiform

Cuboid

Navicular

Head of talus

Medial plantaris nerve

Calcaneus

Lateral plantaris nerve

The foot's structure provides our base and foundation. The average foot contains 26 small bones – each one has a specific job to do. The same is true of the hands, each of which contains 27 bones.

The **Head**

The reflex points for all of the parts of the body that are above the shoulders, including the brain, are found in the toes.

• The brain is represented by the tip of the big toe. The tips of the other toes aid in fine-tuning.

• The pituitary gland reflex is found approximately in the middle of the fleshy part of the big toe of both feet. The reflexes for the sinuses are found in the other four toes, both on the backs and also along the sides of the toes.

• The eye reflex is found at the base of the second and third toes, just below where the toes join the ball of the foot.

• The ear reflex is found at the base of the fourth and fifth toe, just below where the toes join the ball of the foot.

• The Eustachian tube reflex is found just below the web, between the third and forth toes.

• The face is represented by the front of the big toe.

• The teeth and gum reflexes are found on the front of the four small toes.

• The neck reflex is found between the fleshy part of the big toe and the fleshy pad of the ball of the foot.

The toes contain many of the reflexes governing the head and neck area of the body.

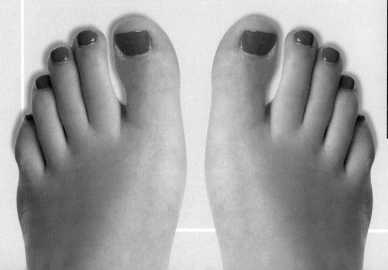

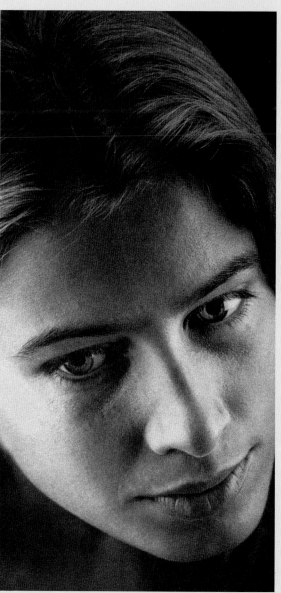

Reflex points for the brain, face, teeth, ears, eyes, mouth, neck and sinuses are all to be found on the toes of the foot.

HEAD REFLEX POINTS

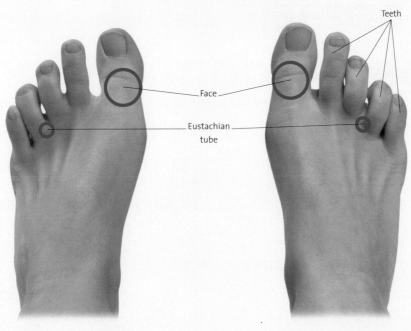

Teeth

Face

Eustachian
tube

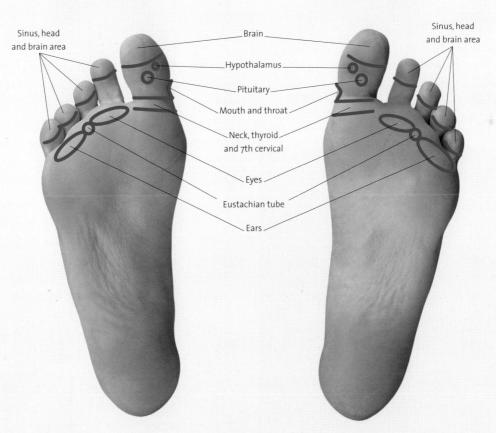

Sinus, head
and brain area

Sinus, head
and brain area

Brain

Hypothalamus

Pituitary

Mouth and throat

Neck, thyroid
and 7th cervical

Eyes

Eustachian tube

Ears

The **Thoracic** and **Upper Abdominal** Area

The ball of the foot contains the reflex points that relate to the thoracic area, and the points relating to the upper abdominal area are on the arch of the foot.

• The shoulder reflex is found at the base of the little toe on the sole, outer side and top of the foot. It extends to about half-way down the fifth metatarsal.
• The lung reflex is found across zones 2 to 5, over the metatarsal bones of the foot. Both the sole and the top of the foot act as a reflex to the lungs. Reflexes for the tracheae, bronchi and oesophagus are found between the big toes and second toes.
• The diaphragm reflex is on the soles of both feet, half-way up the metatarsal bones, across all 5 zones.
• The heart reflex is found in the left foot in zones 2 and 3, just above the diaphragm reflex, even though the heart itself is in zone 1.

• The thyroid reflex is found in zone 1, over the upper part of the ball of the foot. As the thyroid is in the neck, the left half is found in the left foot and the right half in the right foot. The thyroid gland controls the metabolic rate by producing thyroxine. It also produces calcitonin, which increases the uptake of calcium by the bones. The four parathyroid glands are found on the lobes of the thyroid; they produce the parathormone, which regulates the concentration of calcium by causing the bones to release calcium into the body. This knowledge is useful when treating arthritis, osteoporosis and cramp, and metabolic disorders. The parathyroid reflexes are closely linked with the thyroid reflexes. An upper and lower parathyroid reflex will be found in both feet.
• The thymus gland reflex is found in zone 1 in both feet, over the ball of the big toe. The thymus gland is important before puberty in helping to develop the body's immune system. Its exact function in adulthood is unclear.
• The solar plexus reflex is found at the same level as the diaphragm in zone 3. This reflex may be used to induce a relaxed state and is often used at the end of a treatment to leave the patient calm. It is useful for the treatment of hiccups. The solar plexus consists of a network of nerve ganglia and is the nerve supply of the abdominal organs below the diaphragm.

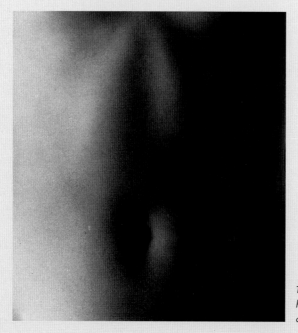

The solar plexus has long been known to have a strong connection with feelings of calmness and well-being.

• The liver reflex is found on the sole of the right foot, between the diaphragm reflex and the waistline, and it fills most of this area, because the liver is the largest and most complex organ in the body. It has many functions, including processing nutrients from the blood, detoxifying the blood, and storing fats and sugars until the body has a need for them. It also produces bile for fat digestion. The bile is stored in the gall bladder. The gall bladder reflex is found in zone 4, in the liver area.

• The stomach reflex is located on the soles of both feet. In the left foot, the reflex occupies zones 1 to 4, while on the right foot it occupies zones 1 to 2. The stomach is to be found between the diaphragm and the waistline.

• The pancreas reflex is similar to the stomach reflex, being found in zones 1 to 4 on the left foot, and zones 1 to 2 on the right foot. It is found between the waistline, running half-way up towards the diaphragm. The pancreas is responsible for secreting insulin and glucagon (thereby acting as an endocrinal gland). These two hormones are responsible for the control of the sugar metabolism, and this reflex is therefore important in the treatment of diabetes. The pancreas also acts as an exocrine gland by excreting digestive juices.

• The spleen reflex is to be found on the left foot between zones 4 and 5, at a similar horizontal level to the stomach.

• The kidney reflexes are found on the soles of both feet, at about waistline level in zones 2 to 3. The right kidney is slightly lower than the left kidney, both in the body itself and in the positioning of the reflexes.

• The adrenal gland reflexes are on the soles of both feet, just above and slightly inside the kidney reflex in zone 2. The adrenal glands consist of an outer cortex which produces steroid hormones. These regulate carbohydrate metabolism and have anti-allergic and anti-inflammatory properties. The cortex surrounds the central medulla. Adrenalin is secreted by the medulla when the body is placed under stressful conditions which give rise to fear or anger.

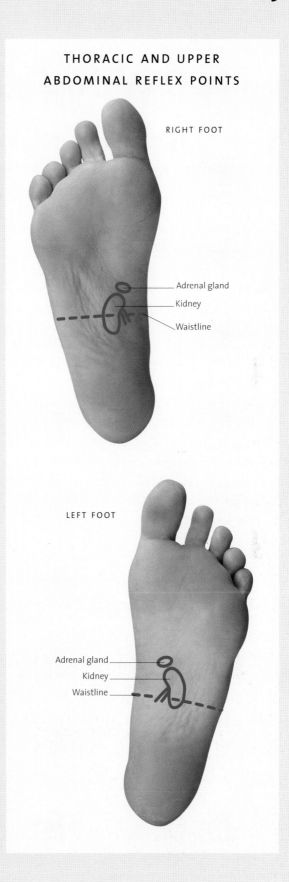

THORACIC AND UPPER ABDOMINAL REFLEX POINTS

RIGHT FOOT

Adrenal gland
Kidney
Waistline

LEFT FOOT

Adrenal gland
Kidney
Waistline

The **Lower Abdominal** Area

Reflex points including the small intestine, the ileo-cecal valve, the appendix, the large intestine, the ureters and the bladder all relate to the lower abdominal area.

• The small intestine reflex is found on the soles of both feet, in between the waistline and pelvic line from zones 1 to 4. The small intestine is a muscular tube about 6–7 metres long. It is divided into three sections. The small intestine is found in the abdomen, doubling back on itself. This is the main area of the digestive tract, where absorption takes place. It leads from the pyloric sphincter of the stomach to the caecum of the large intestine.

• The ileo-caecal valve reflex is found on the right sole, in the line between zones 4 and 5, just above the pelvic line. The valve itself controls the passage of the contents of the small intestine through to the large intestine. It prevents backflow of faecal matter from the large intestine, and controls mucous secretions.

• The appendix reflex is found at the same location as the ileo-caecal valve.

• The large intestine reflexes are found on both feet. On the right foot this begins just above the reflex for the appendix and ileo-caecal valve. It extends upwards (representing the ascending colon), turning just below the waistline to become the transverse colon, which goes across the entire foot, extending to the left foot, turning at the end of zone 5 below the spleen reflex, to become the descending colon. Just above the pelvic line another turn is made into the sigmoid colon; this drops gradually down to the pelvic line at zone 3 to rise in line to the bladder reflex in zone 1, where it ends at the rectum reflex.

The large intestine is a muscular tube about 1.5 metres long. It starts at the ileo-caecal valve, going up the right side of the body (this is the ascending colon) to below the liver, where it bends; this is referred to as the hepatic flexure. The large intestine then passes across the body as the transverse colon. It bends down below the spleen at the splenic flexure to become the descending colon. It continues down the left side of the abdomen, turning toward the central line and becoming the sigmoid colon. This leads to the rectum, which in turn leads to the anus.

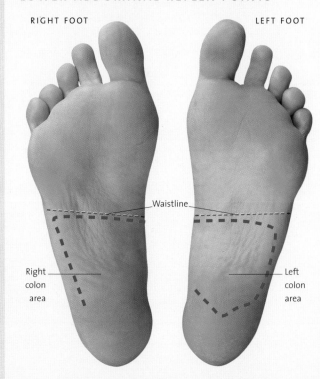

LOWER ABDOMINAL REFLEX POINTS

RIGHT FOOT

LEFT FOOT

Waistline

Right colon area

Left colon area

The partially digested mixture reaches the large intestine as a fluid. By absorbing water and salts the large intestine transforms this fluid mixture into more solid faecal matter that is ready for expulsion. The large intestine also stores the waste faecal matter until it is excreted.

• The ureter reflex is found on the soles of both feet. As may be expected, they link the kidney reflexes to the bladder reflex. This reflex passes from zones 3 to 1. The ureter tubes are about 30 centimetres long. There are two tubes, one from each kidney, which pass downwards through the abdomen and pelvis to the bladder.

• The bladder reflex is found on the soles of both feet, just above the pelvic line. It is often seen as a puffy area in zone 1 on the inner side of the foot.

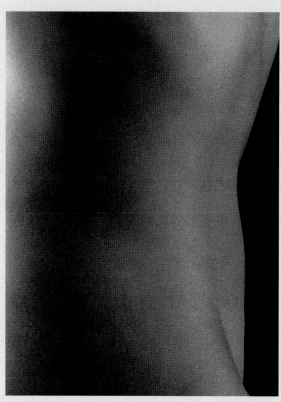

Most of the functions of the digestive and excretory systems take place without our being aware of them, but they can have an important impact on our health.

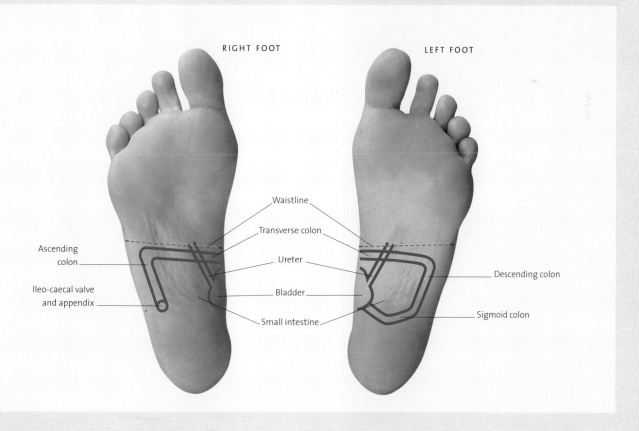

RIGHT FOOT   LEFT FOOT

Waistline

Transverse colon

Ascending colon

Ureter

Descending colon

Ileo-caecal valve and appendix

Bladder

Small intestine

Sigmoid colon

The **Pelvic** Area

Not many organs are represented by reflex points in this area of the foot, but it is important neverthless because six of the main meridians, or energy channels, run through the pelvic area of the body. This means that areas of congestion affecting many organs can be treated here.

• The sciatic nerve reflex is found along the sciatic nerve itself, across the heel, about a third of the way down. It is found on the soles of both feet, and a few centimetres up the ankle on either side of the Achilles tendon. The sciatic nerve is the largest nerve in the body. It arises from the sacral plexus, which is located towards the bottom of the spine, and then passes from the buttock down the back of the leg, dividing behind the knee into two main branches which supply the lower leg.

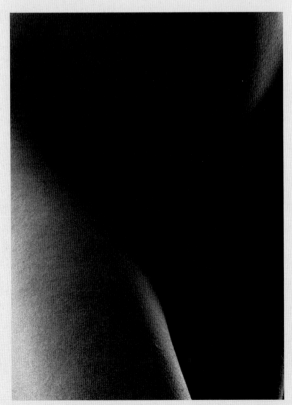

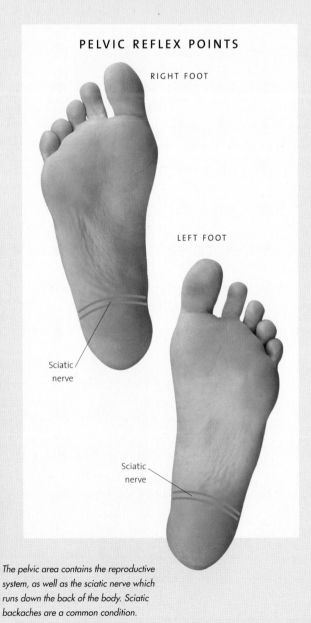

PELVIC REFLEX POINTS

RIGHT FOOT

LEFT FOOT

Sciatic nerve

Sciatic nerve

The pelvic area contains the reproductive system, as well as the sciatic nerve which runs down the back of the body. Sciatic backaches are a common condition.

The **Reproductive** Area

It should be noted that the reflexes for the ovaries (in women) are at the same position on the foot as the reflexes for the testes (in men). Similarly, the reflex that represents the female uterus also represents the male prostate gland.

• The almond-shaped ovaries, one on each side of the uterus, produce ova (eggs), as well as oestrogen and progesterone. The ovary reflexes are on the outer side of both feet, half-way between the ankle-bone and the back of the heel.

• The points for the testes, which produce spermatozoa and testosterone, are as for the ovaries.

• The prostate gland is at the base of the bladder in men, surrounding the urethra. It produces a fluid which aids the transport of semen. The uterus (womb) and prostate reflexes are midway between the ankle-bone and heel, on the outer side of each foot.

• The reflexes for the Fallopian tubes and the seminal vesicle/vas deferens may again be found in the same position on the feet of men and women. They are found across the top of the foot, linking one ankle-bone to the other.

In women, the Fallopian tubes connect the ovaries with the uterus, and so it is logical that, on the foot, the Fallopian tube reflex links the uterus reflex to that of the ovaries. These three areas are usually treated together in reflexology.

In males, the seminal vesicle/vas deferens reflex links the prostate and testes reflexes. Again they should be massaged in conjunction with one another during a treatment. In the body, the seminal vesicles are found next to the prostate, and they store the semen before it is released. The vas deferens are a pair of excretory ducts, which transport the semen from the testes, through the prostate, and into the urethra ready for expulsion.

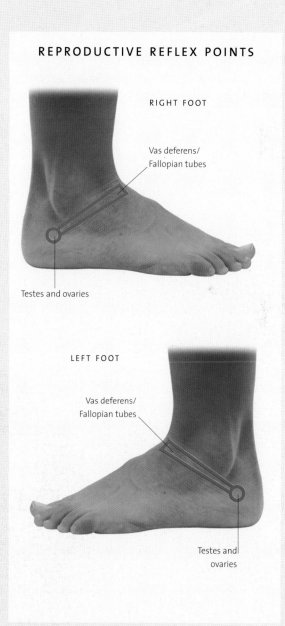

REPRODUCTIVE REFLEX POINTS

RIGHT FOOT

Vas deferens/
Fallopian tubes

Testes and ovaries

LEFT FOOT

Vas deferens/
Fallopian tubes

Testes and
ovaries

The **Spine**

Take a look at the natural curve of your own spine in a mirror, and then look at the arch of your instep. The chances are that the shapes of the curves will mirror each other.

• The spine reflex, as previously mentioned, is found down the inner sides of both feet. The cervical (neck) area is between the top of the side of the big toe, running to the base of the big toe. The thoracic vertebrae are represented by the side of the first metatarsal bone, with the lumbar vertebrae reflex travelling from the waistline of the foot to the inner ankle-bone. The rest of the inside of the foot corresponds to the sacrum and coccyx.

The spine, otherwise known as the backbone or vertebral column, acts as the body's central skeletal support. It carries the weight of the body, acts as protection for the spinal cord, and is also important in movement. In addition, it provides points of attachment for the ribs and back muscles. The spine is made up of 33 vertebrae, and is held in an S-shaped curve by means of the back muscles and ligaments which connect with the vertebrae.

The spine is divided into five sections. Starting from the top, there are: 7 cervical vertebrae (neck area); 12 thoracic vertebrae (back area); 5 lumbar vertebrae (the loins); 5 sacral vertebrae, which are fused in adults (in the pelvis); and 4 or 5 coccyal vertebrae, which again are fused in adults (in the tail). The vertebrae contain disks of cartilage between them, which are held in place by ligaments.

The spine supports the weight of the upper body, protects the spinal cord, promotes movement in the back and centre of the body, and anchors many major nerves.

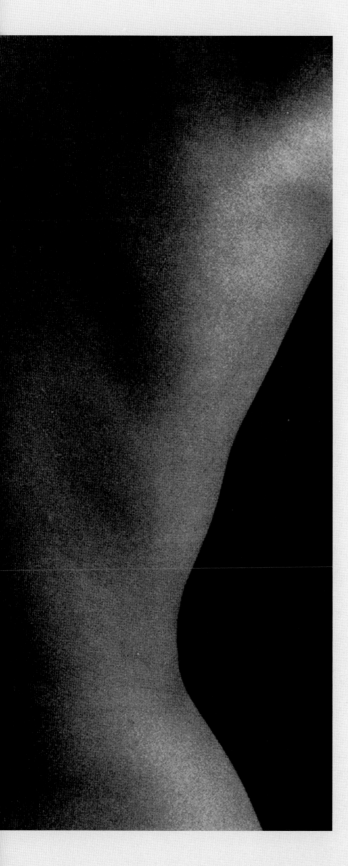

SPINAL REFLEX POINTS

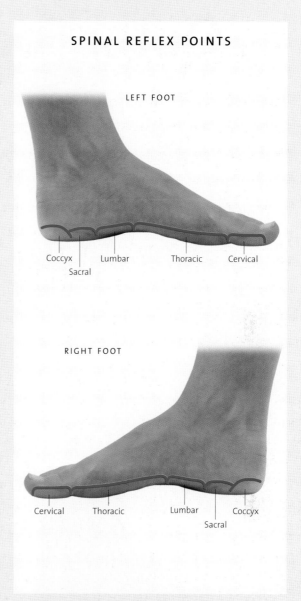

LEFT FOOT

Coccyx | Lumbar | Thoracic | Cervical
Sacral

RIGHT FOOT

Cervical | Thoracic | Lumbar | Coccyx
Sacral

The spinal column encloses the spinal cord, which is a continuation of the brain stem and is the central channel of the nervous system. The spinal cord contains all the nerves that run from the brain to the various parts of the body. Each vertebra has its own pair of spinal nerves, which are named after the place at which they join with the spinal cord. These nerves affect the areas of the body that are on a level with the region of the spine from which they emerge. For example, the thoracic nerves affect the chest, and the lumbar nerves affect the legs and feet.

The **Outer Foot**

It should be noted that different reflexologists and different books vary somewhat in their opinions on the exact locations of the reflexes of the arm, elbow, wrist, hand, leg, knee and foot.

• The upper arm reflex can be found on the outer side of the foot, under the shoulder reflex and the cuboid notch. The elbow reflex is represented by the cuboid notch.

• The pelvic reflex is found over the tarsal bones of both feet. The pelvis is formed by the sacrum and coccyx and the innominate (the large hipbones) at the front and sides. The pelvis contains the bladder, rectum and reproductive organs.

• The knee reflex is found below the pelvis reflex on the outer side of the foot.

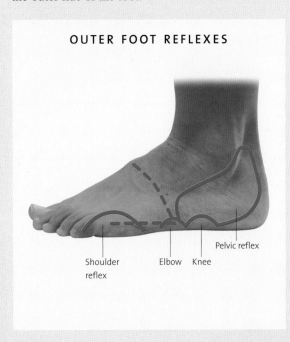

OUTER FOOT REFLEXES

Shoulder reflex   Elbow   Knee   Pelvic reflex

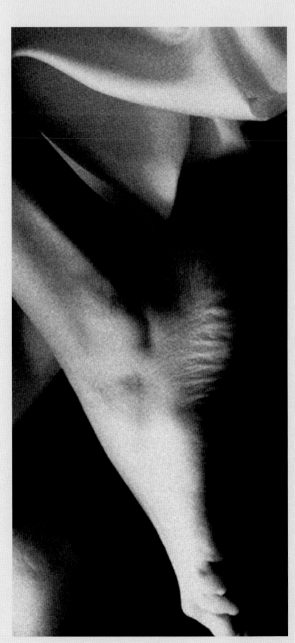

The outer edge of the foot corresponds to the outer parts of the body – limbs, joints and ligaments.

The **Top** of the **Foot**

Reflex points that are to be found on the top of the foot include those for the circulatory system and for the breasts.

• The breast reflex is situated at the top of the foot from behind the toes to about the waistline level.

• The upper lymph node reflexes are found in between the toes. Lymphatic drainage back to the venous system may be stimulated by working these areas on both feet. Work the tops and soles of the foot, between the toes, using a pinching action.

As well as the circulatory system and the breasts, the top of the foot may also be used to treat the meridian lines that traverse it.

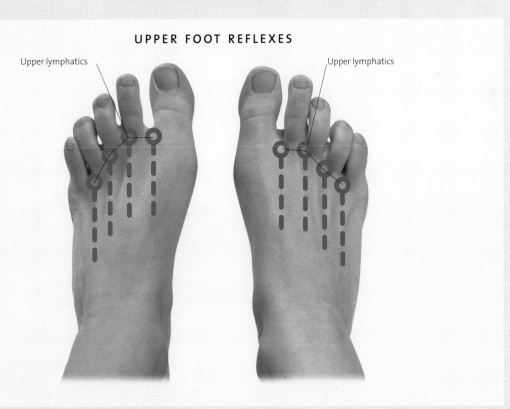

UPPER FOOT REFLEXES

Upper lymphatics

Upper lymphatics

Symptoms and Case Histories

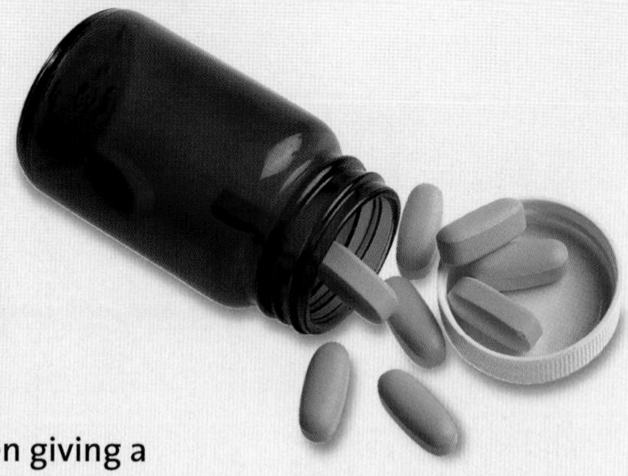

Reflexology is a holistic treatment. This means that, when giving a treatment, it is important to consider the person as a whole, not just the condition or disease being treated.

Reflexologists do not prescribe medicines, but they should be aware of any medication taken by their clients.

A case history of the client should always be taken. This, of course, will tell you about the person's physical health, any medication that they are on, and also if there are any contra-indications present. It will also tell you about their lifestyle, family history and the effect the environment has on them. On further questioning you can find out about the client's past, which may have an effect on their present condition.

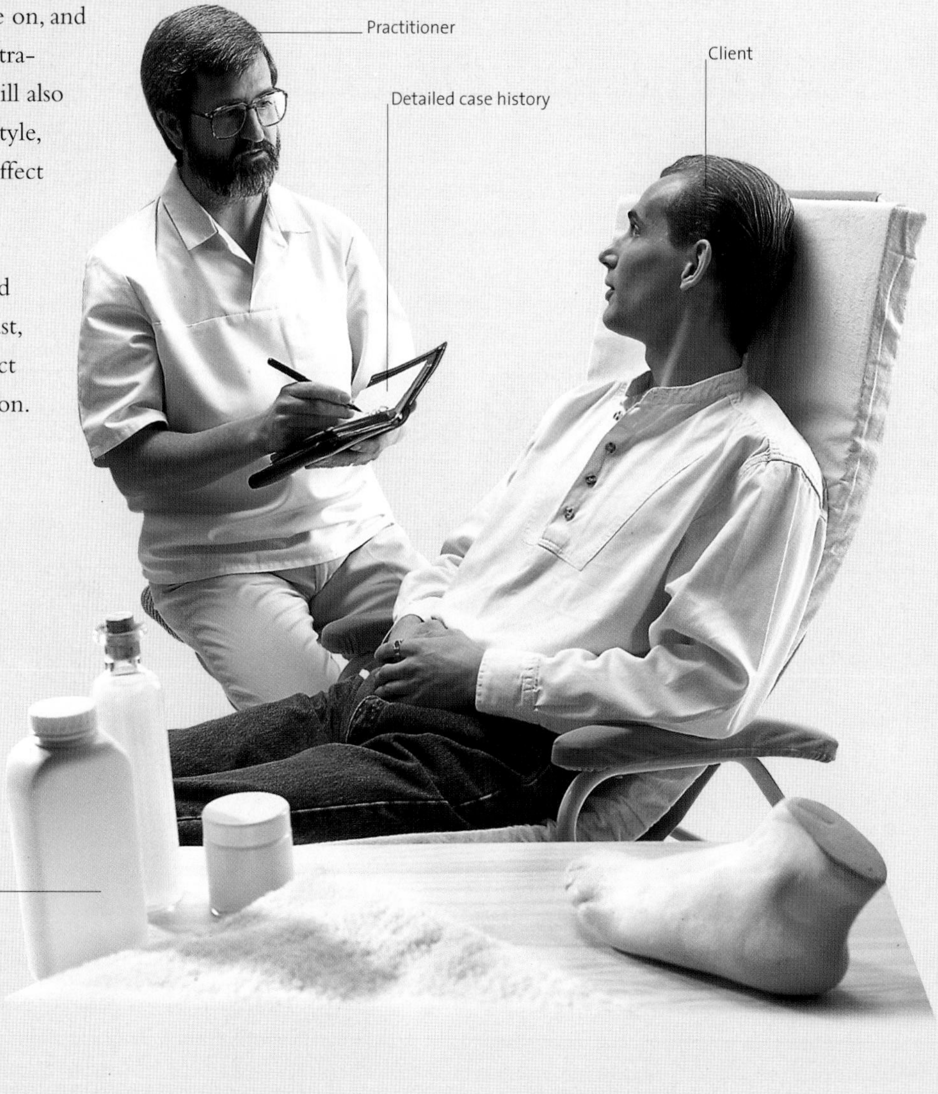

Practitioner

Client

Detailed case history

Responsible practitioners will take detailed case histories from their clients, and will refer any serious complaints to the client's medical doctor.

Foot lotion

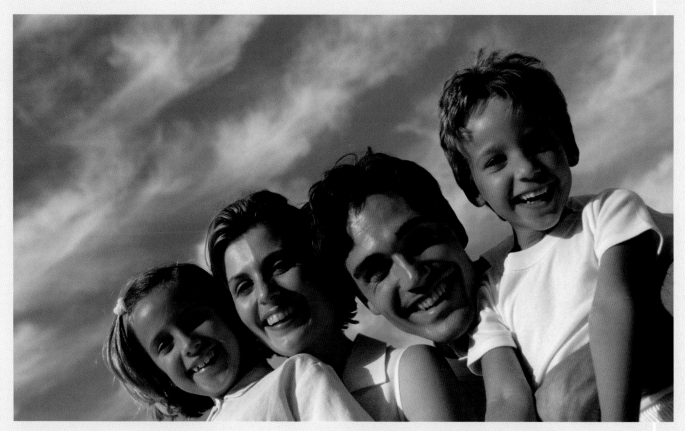

Many chronic conditions or vulnerabilities seem to be passed down through the generations, so it can be very useful to run through the client's family history to build up a full picture.

Reflexology is not a substitute for conventional medical care; rather, it works in tandem with it.

It is worth taking time over the case history of the client. Not only does this process give you valuable information about them, but also allows them to relax in your company and to find out a little bit more about reflexology.

It should be stressed that reflexologists – unless they are licensed physicians – do not practise medicine. This means that they should never try to diagnose a disease, or to prescribe or adjust a client's medication. Responsible reflexologists do not treat specific diseases, although by returning the body to a more harmonious state, a treatment can combat a number of disorders. Reflexologists should always advise their client to see their medical practitioner when necessary.

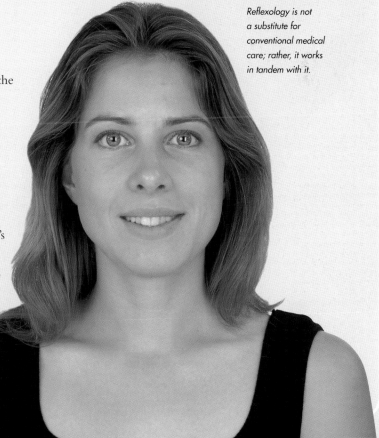

Basic **Techniques**

A reflexology treatment should always be enjoyable and relaxing. Whether the client feels a lot or nothing, the treatment is still effective.

Before treating someone, make sure that your nails are trimmed and your hands clean.

The treatment should not be ticklish, as the massage technique used is too firm to tickle. If the person being treated seems to find it ticklish, try increasing the pressure of your stroke (although be careful not to be too firm, as some reflex points can be tender). Some people feel many sensations while being treated, while others will report feeling almost nothing at all.

BEFORE YOU START

Before you start giving a reflexology treatment, take time to check that the environment is right.
- Ensure you have short fingernails.
- Take the phone off the hook.
- Make sure that the room is heated to a comfortable temperature.
- Check that the couch or chair being used by the client is comfortable. Their lower legs should be supported and possibly raised, with the feet in a comfortable position.
- Shoes and socks should be removed. Any tight-fitting garments should be loosened to allow the energy to flow through the body.

The chair you use should be comfortable for your client, but also ensure that it is at the right height for you.

THE SESSION CAN NOW BEGIN.

The feet can either be washed in a footbath, or cleaned with wet wipes. The client may soak their feet in the footbath while you are doing their case study. If you were giving a home treatment, the client may have washed their feet prior to your arrival.

All feet are different, and a lot of useful information can be picked up by looking at the feet, especially their colour, and checking their temperature. Cold feet that are rather blue or red indicate poor circulation, as does dry skin on the foot. Feet that perspire indicate a glandular imbalance.

A long soak in a foot bath will have the dual effect of cleaning the feet and softening any hard skin, making massage easier.

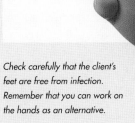

Check carefully that the client's feet are free from infection. Remember that you can work on the hands as an alternative.

Cracks in the soles, calluses, corns or bunions and so on should be noted, together with the area in which they occur; for example, cracks on the heel usually indicate pelvic disorders. Also, consider which zones on the feet these features occur in, and make connections to the relevant body zone. An ingrowing toenail may relate to headaches or migraine; flat feet may indicate a problem with the spine.

Feet that feel tense will inform you that the client is stressed. Limp feet tend to indicate poor muscle tone. If there is puffiness around the ankle, internal problems may be present.

Massage Techniques

After ensuring that the client is not allergic to talcum powder, apply a small amount to the feet. Massage oils make the surface of the foot too slippery for reflexology. Talcum powder gives the right amount of slip and also, as feet do have a tendency to perspire, the talcum powder will keep the feet dry. However, some practitioners prefer not to use talcum powder, and this is also fine.

Only a few, simple tools are needed during the course of a treatment.

The reflexology massage technique is mainly performed with the thumb; right and left thumbs are used at different times. The fingers also have a part to play at various times. The thumb is bent at about 45° and 'walks' along the foot in very small 'steps', doing the 'caterpillar walk' (CW). Each reflex is about the size of a pinhead so, for the treatment to be effective, precision is required. The pressure used should be firm, but not too aggressive. The hands and fingers are also used to support the foot and sometimes to provide leverage.

It takes a while to master the technique; it may take time to build up the necessary strength. Practitioners should check their technique regularly, as they may be at risk from tendonitis.

The client may feel a variety of sensations. On the first session, the client may feel little or no tenderness on the foot. This does not mean that there are no areas of congestion; usually it indicates a blockage in the feet which needs to be freed. Frequently, the feet become more sensitive during subsequent sessions. The tenderness that is felt in the points representing the congested areas will also diminish over the course of treatment. The number of treatments that are needed will depend on the client. Although some pain may be felt on some of the reflexes, the treatment as a whole should not be painful, and should leave the client relaxed and refreshed.

After applying talcum powder to the feet, the feet can be covered with a towel to keep them warm.

This shows the most usual position of the thumb and fingers in reflexology; the thumb is bent at an angle and pressure is applied by the pad, while the fingers support the foot.

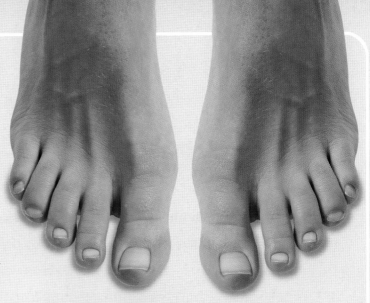

There are relaxation techniques that relax the foot before (and often after) the treatment. The circulation is stimulated, which warms the client's feet and sometimes their whole body. It also allows the client to become accustomed to your touch.

You may choose to relax both feet, and then begin the main treatment; or the right foot can be relaxed and then worked on immediately, followed by the same sequence for the left foot.

Not everybody likes their own feet, and some clients may feel embarrassed about exposing them.

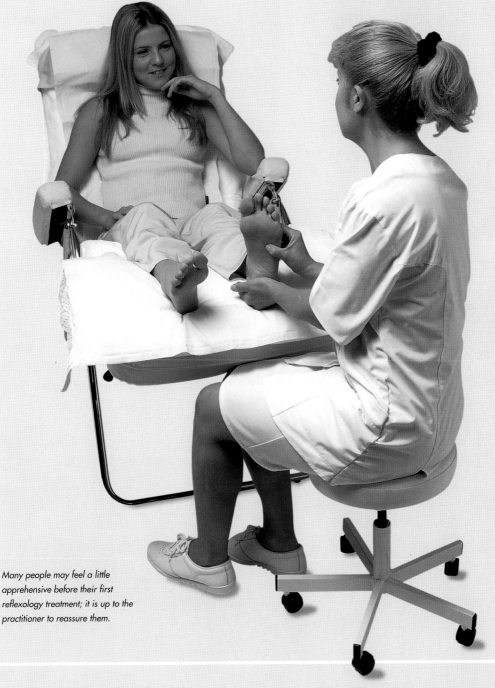

Many people may feel a little apprehensive before their first reflexology treatment; it is up to the practitioner to reassure them.

Relaxing the Foot

As previously discussed, it is advisable to begin each treatment by relaxing the foot using these exercises.

Toe rotation

Starting with the big toe, hold each toe with the finger and thumb of one hand, while the other hand holds the foot. Gently rotate the toe in one direction three times, then rotate it in the opposite direction three times. Give a gentle tug. Then repeat for the other toes, working towards the little toe in sequence.

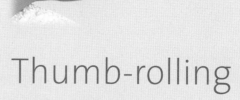

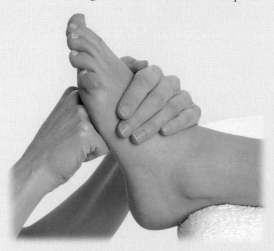

Thumb-rolling

Hold the foot by placing both sets of fingers over the front of the foot with the thumbs on the sole, one above the other, at the bottom of the heel. Firmly place the bottom thumb above the other one. Continue this process until the area from the heel to the base of the toes has been thumb-rolled.

Metatarsal kneading

With one hand holding the foot at the toes, clench the other hand to form a fist. Starting at the fleshy part of the sole just under the toes, use your fist to push against the foot in a kneading motion down the foot to the heel, moving the other hand down at the same time to maintain support of the client's foot. This can be repeated a few times.

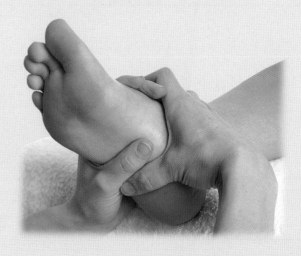

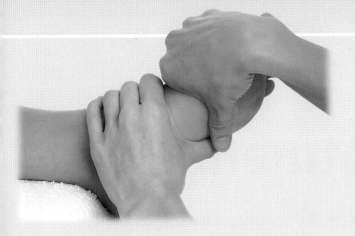

Achilles' tendon stretch

Cup the heel in one hand, and with the other hand grasp the top of the foot near the toes. Pull the toes towards you, allowing the heel to move backwards, then pull the heel towards you, allowing the toes to move backwards. Repeat this a few times.

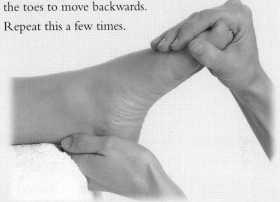

Spinal twist

Place the fingers of both hands side by side, holding the top of the foot by the ankle with the thumbs on the sole, in a position similar to that used when a Chinese burn is given to the wrist. The hand close to the heel is kept still, while the other hand slowly and smoothly rotates the foot back and forth. Ensure that the foot is rotated evenly in both directions.

Repeat this a few times and then edge forward towards the toes, using the same technique. Continue until you reach the toes.

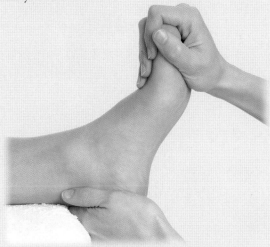

Foot wobbling

Place one palm on each side of the ankle, at right angles to the foot. Keeping the hands and wrists relaxed, rock the foot side to side by gently moving your hands back and forth in opposite directions. Gradually move the hands up from the ankle to the toes so that the whole of the foot is worked on. This technique is good for relaxing the foot and lower leg, and it also aids circulation.

Ankle rotation

Cup the heel in one hand, and with the other hand firmly hold the toes and part of the sole. Keeping your cupped hand still, gently rotate the foot clockwise in complete circles a few times, then anti-clockwise. This technique, as well as being relaxing, also stimulates the reflex that relates to the uterus and the prostate, and the whole of the hip area.

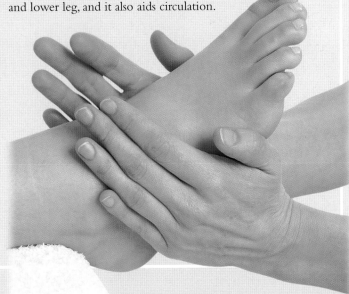

The **Main Treatment**

**Once the feet have been thoroughly relaxed and the client is feeling at ease,
then you will be ready to begin giving the main treatment.**

It is worth asking the client how they feel and what sensations they are experiencing during a treatment. These can be emotional as well as physical. Make sure that the pressure you use is comfortable for the client, not too hard or too soft. I usually check on these things three or four times during a treatment. Sometimes the client will tell you anyway, in which case there is no need to ask! If the client falls asleep, which is quite common during a treatment, don't wake them up to ask.

When the client tells you an area is tender, release the pressure slightly and rework the area. Also, rework the area whenever you feel any blockages. Such blockages may feel like sand under the skin, or like a miniature bubble, rather like those found on bubble-wrap. Keep a note for your records, so that you can compare the state of the reflex the next time a treatment is carried out.

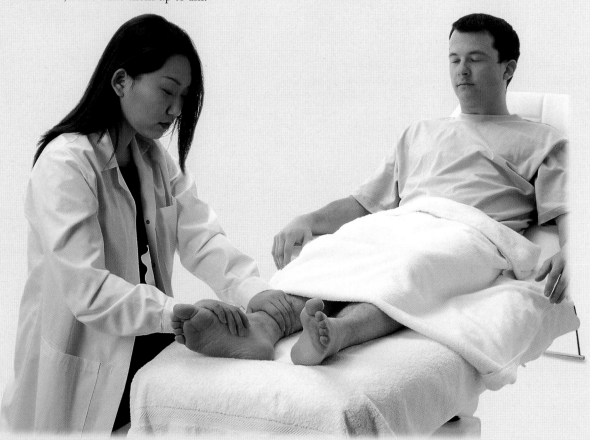

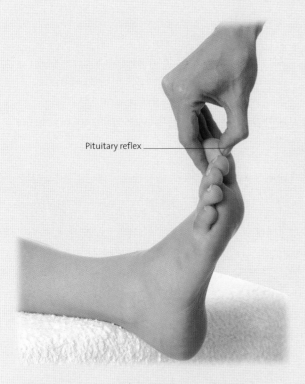

Pituitary reflex

2 CW over the toes starting with the sole of the big toe, walking upwards, then across the face reflex. With the other toes, go up the back and down the front, working towards the little toe in sequence. CW over the tops of the toes in both directions. Be sensitive to what your fingers feel; tenderness is frequently felt while working on these areas. CW over the neck reflex, from the outside of the big toe towards zone 2.

Back of head reflex

1 With the thumb in the bent position as previously described, pinch the hypothalamus reflex by placing the hand over the toes, the fingers over the front of the toe and the thumb over the reflex, and using a pinching, squeezing motion. Repeat for the pituitary reflex.

TIP
Babies respond particularly well to stimulation of these reflexes, although treatments should be light in pressure and short in duration.

Eye and ear reflex

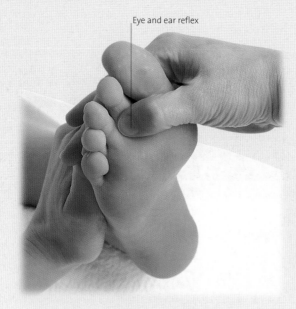

5 Work the shoulder reflex. Start low down on the sole part of the reflex, doing the CW with the thumb, working towards the toes. Then work on the shoulder reflex at the front of the foot, using the index finger to perform the CW. The shoulder reflex is often crunchy, again because of the tension found in this area.

Shoulder reflex

3 CW over the eye and ear reflex in both directions. It helps if you pull back some of the fleshy part of the ball of the foot with one hand while working these reflexes.

Spine reflex

4 Work over the Eustachian reflex, making a pinching and circling motion with the thumb and index finger. Work up and down the spine reflex, using CW. When you reach the heel, slightly increase the level of pressure. Many people find parts of this reflex tender, so remember to ask how your client is feeling, and be sensitive to any areas of congestion. It is worth working the spine reflex more than once, as tension is frequently found at some part of the spine.

6 Work the outer foot. Starting at the base of the little toe, work the arm, elbow, knee and leg reflexes, ending with the hip. Work the cuboid notch in both directions. The hip reflex should also be worked in a criss-cross manner.

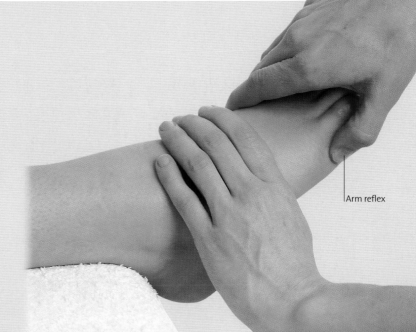

Arm reflex

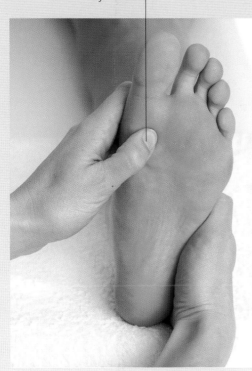

Thymus reflex

8 CW the sole part of the lung reflex, while your left hand thumbs over the diaphragm reflex, with the fingers resting over the front of the foot. Work this reflex both upwards and downwards. Then CW the front part of the foot from zone 5 to zone 1 over the lung reflex.

Lung reflex

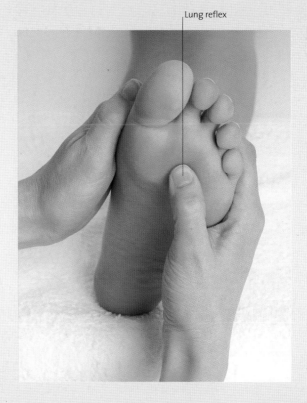

7 Stimulate the thymus, thyroid and parathyroid reflexes thoroughly. The best way to do this it to make a circling motion with the thumb.

9 CW over the line of the diaphragm reflex in both directions with your thumbs, resting your fingers on the front of the foot.

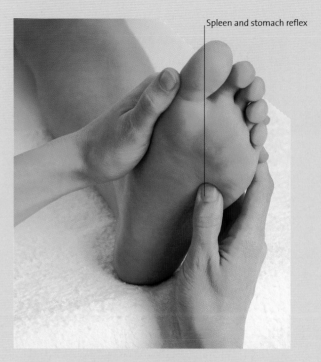

Spleen and stomach reflex

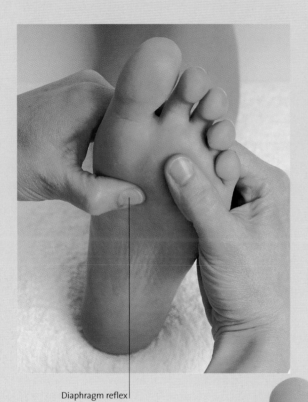

Diaphragm reflex

10 Work the spleen and stomach reflexes by doing the CW across zones 1 to 2.

11 Work the liver reflex by CW in a criss-cross manner. Hook the gallbladder with the index finger and hold it for a few seconds.

Gallbladder reflex

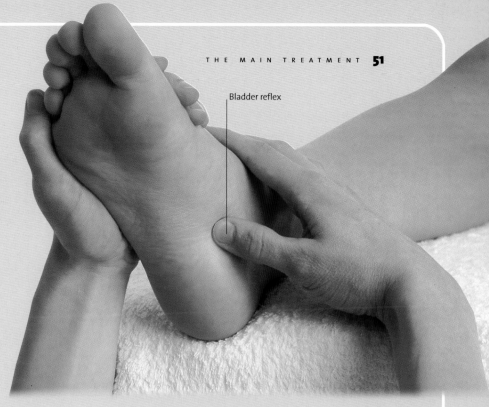

Bladder reflex

TIP

It is useful to remember that the line of the diaphragm reflex also represents the dividing line between the ball and the arch of the foot.

12 Work the small intestine reflex by CW in both horizontal directions.

Small intestine reflex

14 Work the bladder reflex by CW diagonally upwards toward the little toe. The bladder, ureter, kidney and adrenal gland reflexes can be tender, so ask the client how they are during this part of the treatment.

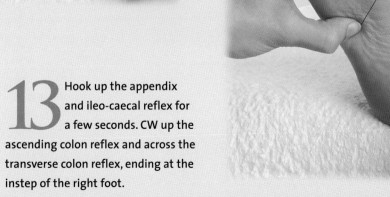

Appendix reflex

13 Hook up the appendix and ileo-caecal reflex for a few seconds. CW up the ascending colon reflex and across the transverse colon reflex, ending at the instep of the right foot.

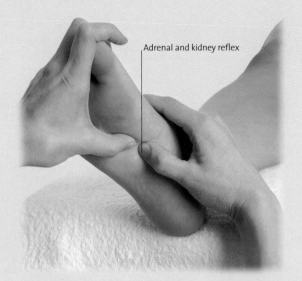

Adrenal and kidney reflex

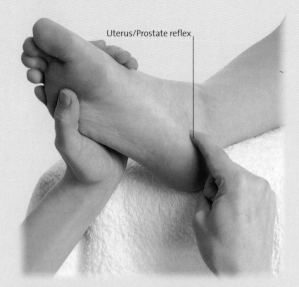

Uterus/Prostate reflex

15 Work up the ureter reflex and the kidney reflex by CW, stimulate the adrenal reflex, then work down the ureter reflex and bladder reflex. Work the bladder reflex two or three times. The kidney and adrenal reflexes can be stimulated together. This is done by placing one thumb on the kidney reflex and the other one on the adrenal reflex, with the two thumbs facing each other. Pull the two thumbs away from one another, and gently massage the reflexes with the thumbs for about 30 seconds.

16 Stimulate the ovary/testes reflex by circling the index finger over the reflex for a few seconds. Then, using two fingers, CW over the Fallopian/vas deferens reflex to the uterus/prostate reflex. Repeat the circling motion over the uterus/prostate reflex for a few seconds, and then stimulate the Fallopian/vas deferens reflex again, finishing at the ovary/testes reflex.

Sciatic nerve reflex

17 CW over the sciatic nerve reflex across the pelvic line near the heel and up the sides of the heel. Then, using the fingers, work up the sciatic nerve reflex on both sides of the ankle, then back down and across the pelvic line again. When doing the heel part, put more pressure on the thumbs to give a slightly harder treatment in this area.

Using all four fingers, CW over the front of the foot starting at zone 5 and CW across the foot to zone 1.

18 Using all four fingers, CW over the front of the foot starting at zone 5 and CW across the foot to zone 1.

20 Massage the lymphatic system reflexes found between each toe. This is done by pinching the web between each of the toes, starting at the big toe and working towards the little toe. After you have pinched the web slowly and firmly, using both your index finger on the top of the foot, and your thumb on the sole of the foot, perform a series of pinches down the metatarsals. Then come back to the web by squeezing the flesh of the foot between your finger and thumb.

Lymph of the groin reflex

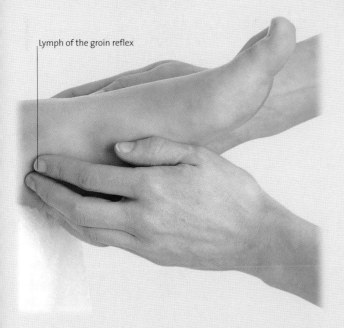

19 Using your fingers, gently massage around the ankle-bone – this is also a reflex to the lymph of the groin. Tenderness here relates to pelvic inflammation.

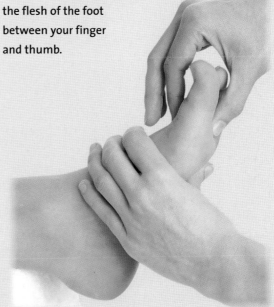

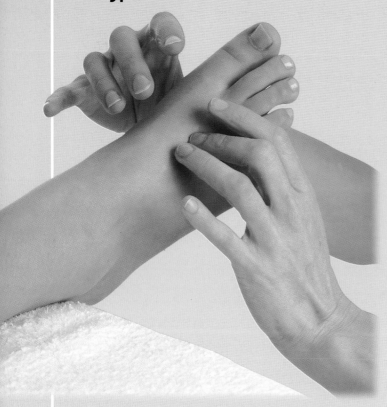

24
Work the small intestine reflex by CW in both horizontal directions.

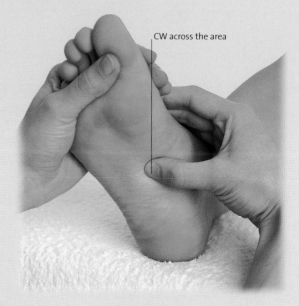

CW across the area

21
Using all your fingers gently tap (as if you were playing the piano) the whole of the front of the foot.

22
Now wrap a towel around the right foot, and start the treatment on the left foot. Use the same massage steps as in the right foot until you finish at the diaphragm reflex.

23
Work the spleen and stomach reflexes by doing the CW across zones 1 to 4.

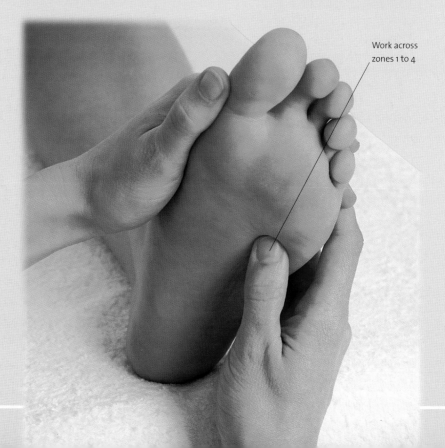

Work across zones 1 to 4

25 CW across the transverse colon reflex, down the descending colon reflex, and along the sigmoid colon, dropping just below the pelvic line at the mid line, then up towards the bladder reflex. Give the rectum reflex a squeeze with the thumb.

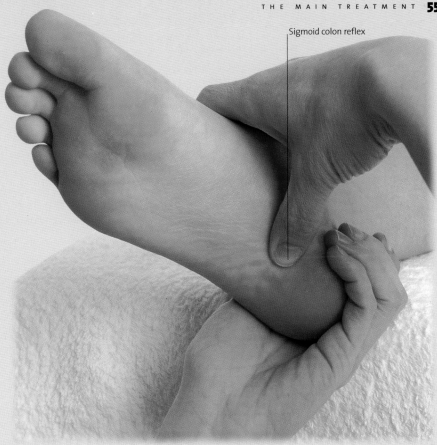

Sigmoid colon reflex

TIP
Allow the client to sit quietly for some time after the treatment, particularly if they have been asleep, as they may be disorientated for a short while.

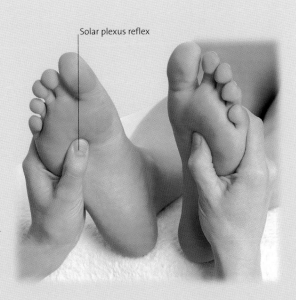

Solar plexus reflex

26 Now work the rest of the left foot in a similar manner to the right foot. When both feet have had the main treatment, the solar plexus relaxation treatment can be given. This relaxation method can also be given at the start of a treatment. The solar plexus is the main storage area for stress, and applying pressure to this area can always bring about a degree of relaxation.

This technique should be applied to both feet simultaneously. Take the right foot in the left hand, and the left foot in the right hand. The fingers should be wrapped around the side of the foot, with the thumbs over the solar plexus reflex. Ask the client to inhale slowly while you press on the solar plexus reflex, and exhale as you release the pressure. Do not lose contact with the foot while you are doing this. Repeat the process about three times.

Reactions Following a Treatment

Once the treatment has finished, the client should feel relaxed and perhaps warmer, because the stimulation of the blood circulation. Sometimes, however, the client may feel cold – this is because of the toxins leaving the body.

I n order for the body to heal itself, it has to get rid of toxic substances. The severity of the healing crisis depends upon the person and their imbalances. So that the client does not have too strong a healing crisis, it is always best to give a gentle first treatment, and to observe the client and their reactions before the second one is given, which can be better tailored to their needs.

Most forms of disease will have been building up over a period of time. It is, therefore, unrealistic to expect an instantaneous improvement.

Ask your client how they are feeling after the treatment has finished. Have a blanket or some warm towels to hand in case they are feeling cold.

People are often surprised after a treatment that stimulating points on the feet can have such a dramatic effect across the body.

COMMON REACTIONS

Here are some of the more common reactions that may occur.

• Perhaps the most common is that the client has a very good night's sleep.

• The rate of urination may increase. The colour and smell may also change.

• The client may get a cold.

• Some people experience a headache. If this does occur, it is best not to take any medication to try to suppress it.

• Suppressed past conditions could flare up.

These are all positive reactions, and show that the body is trying to heal itself. The healing crisis is usually short-lived, leaving the person with a heightened feeling of well-being.

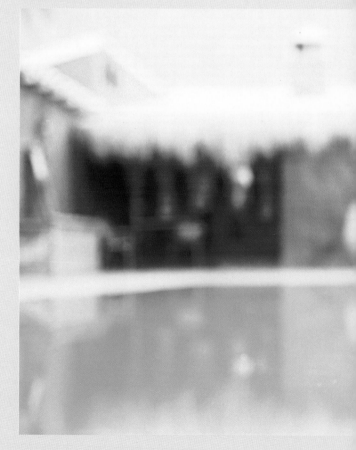

NUMBER OF TREATMENTS REQUIRED

Every client is different, so it is not possible to predict the exact number of sessions required. Serious diseases usually take longer to treat than minor ones. Disorders that have been present for a long time again usually take longer than those that have been present for only a short time. Older people usually take longer than younger people do. A lot, however, depends on the individual person and their attitude.

For all diseases, a course of treatment is recommended even if the symptoms appear to go after the first treatment. The course of treatment will help to balance the body's systems, which will in turn help to prevent a recurrence of the disorder.

For the majority of disorders, a course of six to eight weekly sessions is recommended. Usually some sort of improvement should occur after about three sessions. If after four sessions there does not seem to be any noticeable change in the patient, then perhaps reflexology is not going to be of help in their case. However, there are few people who do not benefit in some way from reflexology. Even if the disorder is not completely cured, the person often feels more relaxed, or better in themselves.

PRECAUTIONS

As previously stated, most disorders will benefit from a reflexology treatment. There are some conditions, however, for which reflexology is unsuitable. These include the following.

• Conditions requiring surgery.

• Lymphatic cancer.

• Early pregnancy (under 16 weeks), or pregnancies where the woman has a history of miscarriage.

• Some of the more serious circulatory problems, such as phlebitis.

• Deep-vein thrombosis.

• Serious cases of fungal or viral foot infections, such as athlete's foot (in this case a reflexology treatment can be done on the hands).

The following conditions can be treated with reflexology, but great care should be taken. If you are unsure about how to treat any of the following disorders, then do not treat.

• Heart conditions. Here, care should be taken not to over-stimulate the heart. Usually a much gentler treatment is given.

• Epilepsy. In this case, care should be taken with the brain, spinal cord and eyes.

• Diabetes.

Almost everyone will benefit from a course of reflexology, but a good practitioner will know which conditions not to treat.

Diseases and
their Associated Reflex Areas

The mind is very powerful, and has the capacity to act on every cell in the body. Most diseases are a direct result of people's lifestyles, actions or thoughts, and it is important that the sufferer takes an active, positive role in the treatment of their condition.

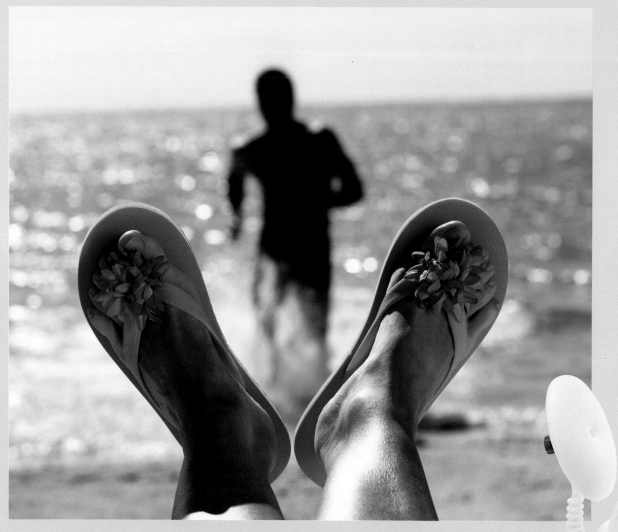

*Holisitc therapies encourage patients to
take responsibility for their own well-being
by adopting healthy lifestyles.*

H ere are some of the more common health problems seen by the reflexologist. It is important to remember, as with many holistic treatments, that even if a specific condition is being treated, a full-body treatment should still be given to ensure the body is correctly balanced. Obviously some areas will require more input than others when treating certain conditions.

Direct reflex (DR) relates to the main body area or areas involved in the condition.

Associated reflex (AR) is an area of the body that may be involved in, or aid in treating, a particular condition.

This section is intended only as a guide. Reflexologists do not diagnose diseases or prescribe; we leave that to the medical profession.

The reflexologist will work with the patient in treating the disease or condition. In order for this to work, the patient must be willing to 'let go' of chronic conditions.

Relexologists are not medical practitioners, and should never attempt to diagnose.

COMMON DISEASES

RESPIRATORY PROBLEMS
Asthma, Sinusitis and Catarrh, Bronchitis.

HEART, BLOOD AND CIRCULATORY PROBLEMS
Angina, Hypertension, Hypotension, Poor circulation.

DIGESTIVE PROBLEMS
Constipation, Gastritis and Ulceration, Gallstones, Heamorrhoids and Piles, Hiatus Hernia, Irritable Bowel Syndrome and Colitis, Liver Problems.

RERPRODUCTIVE PROBLEMS
Heavy Periods, Painful Periods, Pre-menstrual Syndrome, Menopausal Syndrome, Prostate Problems.

ACHES AND PAINS/GENERAL
Gout, Sprains and Strains, Arthritis and Rheumatism, Headaches, Migraine, Colds and Influenza.

EARS, EYES, MOUTH AND THROAT
Earache and ear disorders, Tonsillitis, Sore throat, Conjunctivitis and Blepharitis.

SKIN AND HAIR PROBLEMS
Eczema, Psoriasis, Acne

ALLERGIES
Hay Fever, Urticaria

NERVOUS DISORDERS
Insomnia, Anxiety and Depression

Respiratory Problems

Repiratory problems regularly observed by reflexologists include colds, coughs, bronchitis, emphysema and asthma. These conditions may be associated with smoking, climatic conditions, air pollution, or common bacterial or viral infections.

ASTHMA

This is now a common condition. It is characterized by wheezing and coughing, as the bronchi go into spasm. Asthma can be associated with allergic reactions (for example, hay fever, air pollution or allergy to dust mites). It can also be an inherited condition.

Key symptoms

• Wheezing and difficulty in breathing.
• A feeling of tightness in the chest.
• During an attack, the sufferer has to struggle for air.

DR: Lungs and bronchi.
AR: Diaphragm, solar plexus, cervical and thoracic part of the spine, all the glands (especially the adrenals), ileo-caecal valve, large intestine and heart.

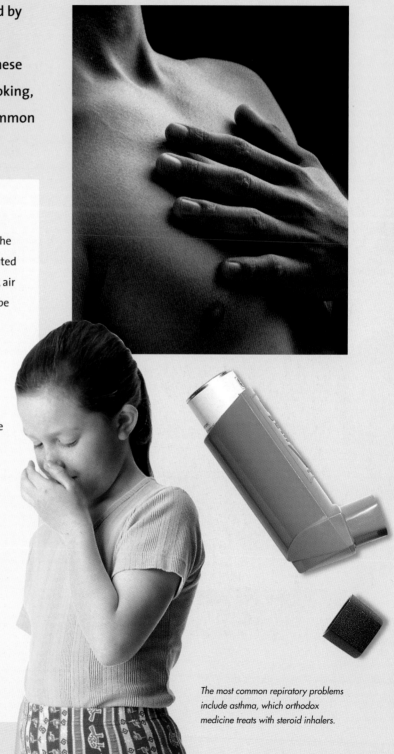

The most common repiratory problems include asthma, which orthodox medicine treats with steroid inhalers.

SINUSITIS AND CATARRH

This is an over-production of mucus from the respiratory membranes, which leads to congestion in the sinus area. Sinusitis occurs when inflammation or infection is present in the sinus cavities.

Key symptoms

• Congestion, which may lead to headaches and earaches.
• The nose may run.
• With sinusitis, a slight temperature is present, which could rise as the infection proceeds.

DR: Big toe, sinuses, and eyes.
AR: Adrenal glands, ileo-caecal valve, large intestine and upper lymphatics.

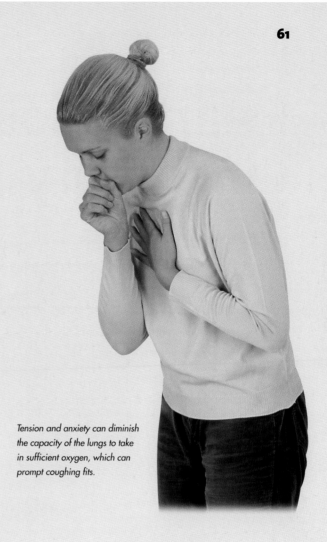

Tension and anxiety can diminish the capacity of the lungs to take in sufficient oxygen, which can prompt coughing fits.

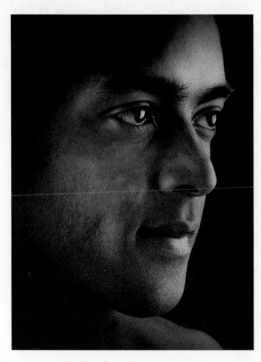

People with a tendency to respiratory infections need to eat plenty of garlic, as well as ensuring that they are getting lots of vitamin C in their diet.

BRONCHITIS

This occurs when the bronchi become inflamed. This can be because of an infection.

Key symptoms

• High temperature.
• A cough that brings up phlegm.
• Wheezing.
• Chest pains and breathlessness.

DR: Lungs and bronchi.
AR: Diaphragm, solar plexus, lymphatics, large intestine, ileo-caecal valve and adrenal glands.

Heart, Blood and Circulatory Problems

These conditions may have serious health implications and should always be referred to a medical doctor. However, reflexology can have a beneficial effect, especially on the circulation.

ANGINA

This is a condition in which there is an insufficient supply of blood to the heart muscles.

Key symptoms

• Short sharp pain experienced in the heart and/or chest area, due to the lack of blood and oxygen in the heart muscles.
• Pain may be felt in the shoulder and/or down the left arm.
• Similar symptoms to heart attacks, but milder.

DR: Heart and lung.
AR: Cervical and thoracic part of the spine, solar plexus, diaphragm, adrenal glands, sigmoid colon.

An efficiently functioning heart is essential for good circulation and can be maintained through exercise, proper nutrition and relaxation.

HYPERTENSION
HIGH BLOOD PRESSURE

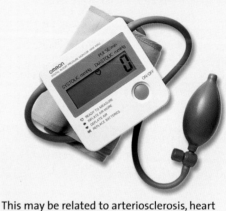

This may be related to arteriosclerosis, heart disorders and liver problems. It can be an inherited condition.

Key symptoms

• Sustained rise in blood pressure above the normal level.
• Headaches, dizziness or fainting spells.
• Eye problems.

DR: Heart.
AR: Big toe, pituitary, solar plexus, diaphragm, adrenals and kidneys.

HYPOTENSION
LOW BLOOD PRESSURE

Some doctors do not feel this condition to be serious, but if the systolic reading (the higher of the two numbers) is consistently below 110 mmHg, they should be informed.

Key symptoms

• Dizziness and/or fainting spells.
• General tiredness and feeling weak.
• Palpitations.

DR: Heart.
AR: Big toe, solar plexus, diaphragm, adrenals and kidneys.

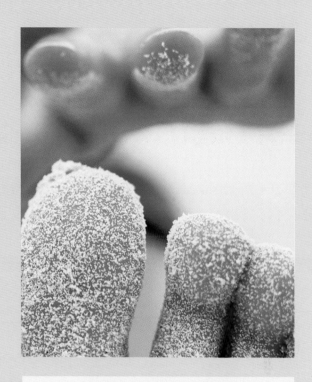

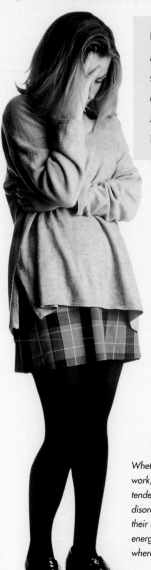

Whether at home or at work, people with a tendency to circulation disorders need to monitor their health, conserve energy, and reduce stress wherever possible.

POOR CIRCULATION

This is usually not a major problem, but it can be a sign of a more serious heart condition.

Key symptoms

• Very cold hands and feet.
• Chilblains may occur.
• Frequently feeling cold.

DR: Heart, direct massage to zone related areas.
AR: Pituitary, adrenals, lungs, liver and intestines.

CAUTION

All heart conditions must be treated with extreme care so that the heart is not over-stimulated.

Digestive
Problems

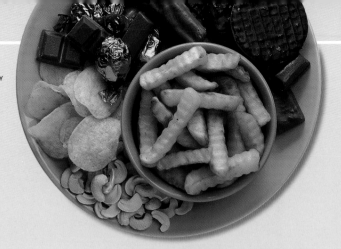

In the West the average diet is so full of saturated fats, and so much in excess of our body's needs, that digestive disorders are very common.

Nuts and chocolate contain some useful vitamins and minerals, but should be eaten in small quantities. Fried foods are best avoided.

CONSTIPATION

Constipation may be associated with poor diet, and a change in the diet may bring about normal bowel movement. Constipation may also be the result of sluggish digestion or muscle tone, and sometimes of stress or nervous tension. it can also be a symptom of other conditions – such as excess iron in the diet or pregnancy – or be the result of taking certain medicines.

Key symptoms

• Lack of bowel movement for at least 24 hours.
• Difficulty in passing stools.
• Low abdominal pain.

DR: Large intestine (pay particular attention to the sigmoid colon, splenic flexure and hepatic flexure), the ileo-caecal valve.
AR: Solar plexus, small intestine, liver, gallbladder, adrenal glands, lower spine.

GASTRITIS AND ULCERATION

Gastritis is inflammation of the stomach lining, which can lead to ulcers, open sores on the bodily surface. Ulcers can occur in the digestive tract – stomach ulcers (gastric ulcers) and small intestine ulcers (duodenal ulcers) are common. Ulcers may be due to dietary factors such as food intolerance, or bacterial or viral infection.

Key symptoms

• Heartburn and the taste of acid in the mouth.
• In acute gastritis there may be persistent vomiting.
• Abdominal pain.

DR: Stomach (gastric ulcer) and small intestine (duodenal ulcer).
AR: Solar plexus, diaphragm and adrenal glands.

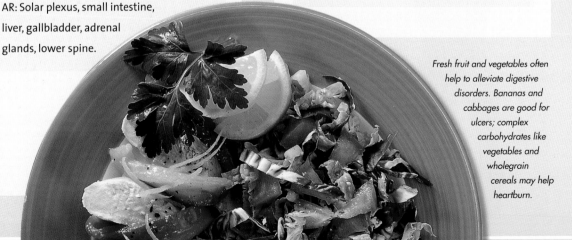

Fresh fruit and vegetables often help to alleviate digestive disorders. Bananas and cabbages are good for ulcers; complex carbohydrates like vegetables and wholegrain cereals may help heartburn.

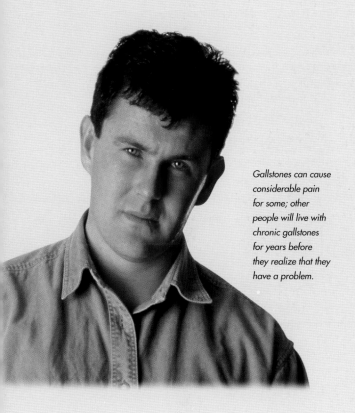

Gallstones can cause considerable pain for some; other people will live with chronic gallstones for years before they realize that they have a problem.

HAEMORRHOIDS PILES

These are anal varicose veins, which can result from persistent straining and/or constipation. They are associated with poor muscle tone.

Key symptoms
• Purple or dark red fleshy lumps within the lining of the anus.
• Bleeding on passing stools.
• Itching or pain around the anus.

DR: Anus/rectum.
AR: Solar plexus, diaphragm, adrenal glands, the large intestine (particularly the sigmoid colon) and the lower spine.

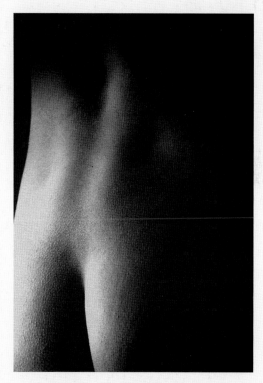

Bowel disease is now one of the major causes of death in the West. Clients should be encouraged to report any sudden changes in excretory habits to their doctor.

GALLSTONES

This is a painful condition. The stones, which are often caused by excess dietary fats, consist mainly of cholesterol and bile pigments, and are found in the gallbladder. If the stones are not too large, it is possible for them to be passed down the bile duct into the small intestine and discharged from the body. Large gallstones may need to be removed by surgery.

Key symptoms
• A yellow colouration (jaundice).
• Severe pain.
• Floating stools.

DR: gallbladder.
AR: Bile duct, liver, solar plexus, thyroid and adrenal glands.

HIATUS HERNIA

A hernia occurs when part of an organ or tissue protrudes through a weak area in the surrounding tissues. A hiatus hernia occurs when the stomach protrudes through the oesophageal opening in the diaphragm and into the chest.

Key symptoms
- Pain.
- Indigestion.
- There may be difficulty in swallowing.

DR: Stomach and diaphragm.
AR: Solar plexus and adrenals.

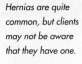

Hernias are quite common, but clients may not be aware that they have one.

IRRITABLE BOWEL SYNDROME AND COLITIS

This is more common in younger and middle-aged women than in men. There are various symptoms, linked to food intolerance, stress, nervousness or an infection.

Key symptoms
- Often a recurring problem.
- Irregular bowel movement with combinations of diarrhoea and constipation.
- 'Rabbit dropping' type stools with mucus.
- Cramp-like pains in the abdomen.
- Bloating and flatulence.

DR: The intestines and rectum.
AR: Solar plexus and adrenals.

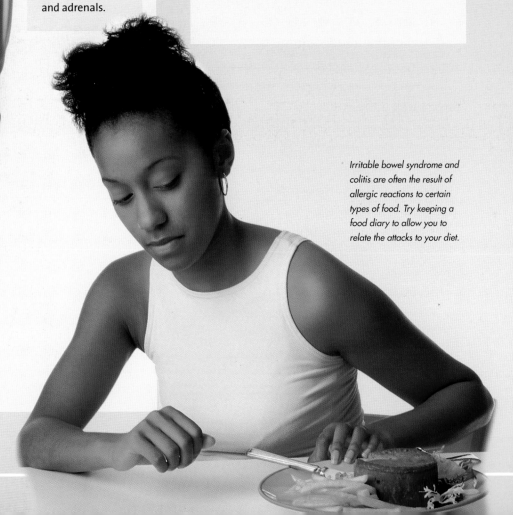

Irritable bowel syndrome and colitis are often the result of allergic reactions to certain types of food. Try keeping a food diary to allow you to relate the attacks to your diet.

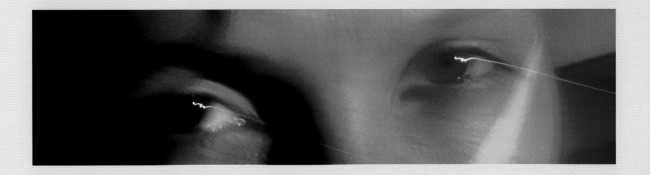

LIVER PROBLEMS

Liver problems are commonly due to excess alcohol, the Western diet with
its high fat content, and the stresses and strains of modern life.

Key symptoms.

- Jaundice.
- Feeling angry.
- Abdominal bleeding.
- Red, itching palms.

- Sore itching eyes.
- Small red abdominal spots.
- Menstrual disorders.
- May suffer frequently from
constipation.

DR: Liver, gallbladder.
AR: Lower back, solar plexus,
eyes, intestines and all glands.

CYSTITIS

This is a infection of the bladder, usually caused
by bacteria. This condition is more common in
women as the urethra is shorter than it is in men.
It is a common problem during pregnancy.

Key symptoms

- Frequent need to pass water.
- Burning sensation when passing water.
- Only small amounts of urine are passed,
and this may be foul-smelling or cloudy, or
contain blood.
- Fever may be present.
- There may be a dull ache in the abdomen.

DR: Kidneys, ureter, bladder and urethra.
AR: Adrenal glands, lymphatics, and lower
spine.

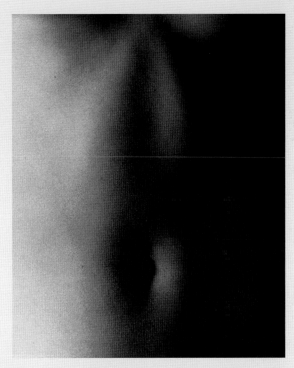

*A common self-help method for cystitis is drinking
plenty of fluid. However, if you are suffering
from recurring attacks, see your doctor to rule
out a more serious condition.*

Reproductive Problems

Disorders of the reproductive system include menstrual disorderers and pelvic inflammatory disease in women. In men, the most common disorder involves the prostate gland in older men.

HEAVY PERIODS
MENORRHAGIA

This occurs when blood loss is abnormally heavy. There can be many causes, including fibroids, having an IUD, endometriosis, pelvic infections, and the run-up to the menopause.

Key symptoms
• Flooding and excessive clots may occur.
• Interferes with normal life.
• The menstrual cycle may be less than 28 days, or the period may last longer than seven days.

DR: Ovaries, fallopian tubes and uterus.
AR: Pituitary, thyroid gland, adrenals, lower back, pelvic area, and lymphatics (if an infection is involved).

Painful periods are quite common, and they can cause a lot of misery for some.

PAINFUL PERIODS
DYSMENORRHOEA

This problem can have a number of causes, including hormonal imbalance, fibroids, pelvic infections and stress.

Key symptoms
• Pain in the lower abdomen or lower back which can vary from a sharp pain or a dull ache to cramp-like pains. These pains can spread down the thighs and legs.
• Bloating may occur in the abdomen.
• Headaches, sweating, diarrhoea and a sensation of nausea may occur.

DR: Ovaries, fallopian tubes and uterus.
AR: Pituitary, thyroid gland, adrenals, lower back, pelvic area, and lymphatics (if an infection is involved).

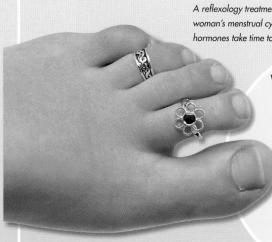

A reflexology treatment may disrupt a woman's menstrual cycle, as the hormones take time to adjust.

CAUTION
When giving female clients a reflexology treatment, extra care should be taken in matters concerning the reproductive organs. Women who are in the first third of their pregnancy, and those who have a history of miscarriage, should be treated with extreme care. If you are at all unsure, do not treat.

PRE-MENSTRUAL SYNDROME

This is usually associated with hormonal imbalance.

Key symptoms

• Emotional.

• Irritable, angry and/or tearful.

• Clumsy.

DR: Ovaries, fallopian tubes and uterus.
AR: Pituitary, thyroid gland, adrenals, lower back, pelvic area.

Reflexology can ease the pain caused by an enlarged prostate gland.

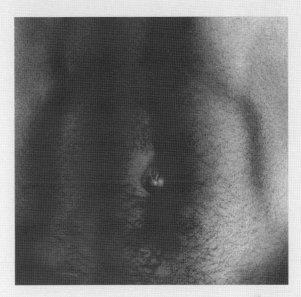

MENOPAUSAL SYNDROME

This is associated with the hormonal changes that usually occur in women who are around 50 years of age.

Key symptoms

• Hot flushes and sweating.

• Mood swings and tearfulness.

• Irregular menstruation, both in terms of the length of the menstrual cycle and the flow of bleeding.

• Vaginal dryness.

• Forgetfulness.

DR: Pelvic area, ovaries, fallopian tubes and uterus.
AR: Pituitary, thyroid gland, adrenals, lower back.

When a woman reaches menopause her hormonal balance changes radically.

PROSTATE PROBLEMS

The more common problems associated with the prostate are infection of the prostate gland, which is more common in younger men, and the enlargement of the gland, which generally occurs in older men.

Key symptoms

• Frequently needing to pass water

• Burning pain when passing water

• Finding it difficult to pass water and dribbling when doing so

• Lower back pain

• The testes may be inflamed

DR: Prostate and testes
AR: Pituitary, thyroid, parathyroid, adrenal glands, kidneys, ureter, bladder, lower back, and lymphatics (if an infection is involved)

Aches and Pains

Some conditions involve chronic pain, which can be difficult to deal with. Other painful conditions are of a limited duration.

ARTHRITIS AND RHEUMATISM

There are two main types of arthritis. Osteoarthritis occurs when the cartilage between the joints wears away. This usually occurs in the knees, hips, neck or spine, though the fingers and thumbs may also be affected. There is pain and swelling of the joints. Rheumatoid arthritis (RA) occurs when the joints become inflamed and painful. The sufferer, who is often female, feels generally unwell. Rheumatoid arthritis requires professional treatment.

Key symptoms

• Stiffness and pain in the joints.

• Bony swellings or deformed joints.

• Hot or burning joints (RA).

• Joints making creaking sounds when moved.

> DR: Joints and areas directly affected.
> AR: Pituitary, parathyroid glands, kidneys and solar plexus.

GOUT

Associated with the build-up of uric acid in the joints. This condition is frequently associated with dietary excess.

Key symptoms

• Swollen and very painful joints, often in the toes or feet.

> DR: Area where condition is present.
> AR: Kidney and adrenal glands reflex.

SPRAINS AND STRAINS

Injuries to joints and muscles, including back strains.

Key symptoms

• Pain following injury or exertion.

• Swollen joints or limbs.

• Bruising may or may not be present.

> DR: Area affected.
> AR: Kidneys, adrenals and lymphatics.

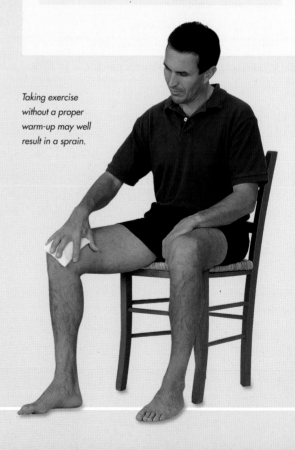

Taking exercise without a proper warm-up may well result in a sprain.

HEADACHES

These may be caused by stress, tension, neck problems, sinus congestion, eye trouble, allergies, and hormonal changes (especially in women).

Key symptoms

• Pain in the head area.

DR: All of the head.

AR: Spine, diaphragm, solar plexus, all the glands and all the toes.

MIGRAINE

This is a severe headache, which can be associated with stress, menstrual cycle, food sensitivity, or pollutants. The symptoms may last for a few minutes to several days if left untreated.

Key symptoms

• Severe pain in the head area.

• Visual disturbances sometimes occur.

• Sensitivity to noise and light.

• Feeling sick or being sick.

• Pins and needles may be felt in the arms and the legs.

DR: All of the head.

AR: Spine, diaphragm, solar plexus, all the glands and all the toes.

Certain foods, including cheese, chocolate and red wine, may trigger a migraine for some.

COLDS AND INFLUENZA

These are usually brought about by viral or bacterial infections, and are often associated with stress, fatigue, depression and extremes of temperature.

Key symptoms

• Fever.

• One or more of the following: cough, cold and/or sore throat.

• Muscle pain and/or headache.

DR: Chest/lung, all head reflexes.

AR: Adrenals, pituitary, intestines, lymph systems and all toes.

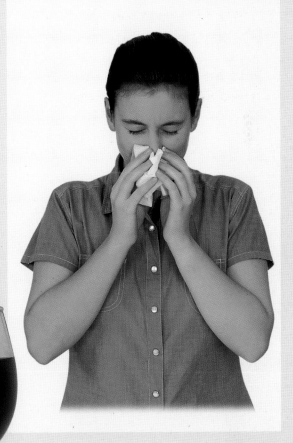

Ears, Eyes, Mouth and Throat

Some people have their tonsils removed in childhood, but for others the problems continue.

A wide range of painful complaints can afflict these parts of the body.

EARACHE AND EAR DISORDERS

Earache is often associated with infection, for example the common cold. Tinnitus occurs when internal 'noises' of various intensities are heard by the client.

Key symptoms

• Pain, often severe in one or both ears, sometimes accompanied by a fever (earache).

• Ears feel blocked and may have a waxy discharge (earache).

• Buzzing or ringing sounds (tinnitus).

• If the inner ear is infected, nausea.

DR: Ears.
AR: All toes, Eustachian tube, neck, cervical spine, solar plexus, upper lymphatics and the adrenal glands.

Earaches and associated conditions are common in children, and are often caused by infection.

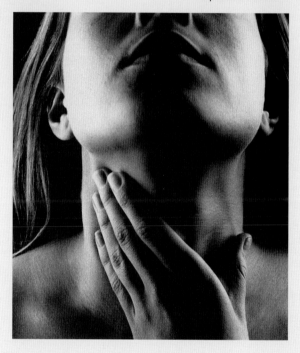

TONSILLITIS

This is inflammation of the tonsils, causing them to swell and go red. This is usually a viral or a bacterial infection.

Key symptoms

• Very sore throat, and the neck may be very tender.

• Red enlarged tonsils, which may have white or yellow spots (pus discharge).

• Finding it hard to swallow.

• Fever.

DR: Neck and cervical spine.
AR: All toes, lymph system and adrenals.

Most common eye conditions, like conjunctivitis, will be eased by reflexology.

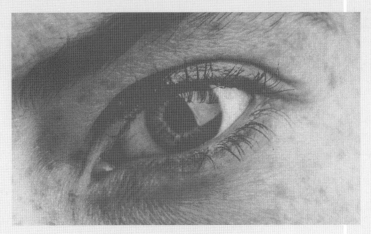

SORE THROAT

This may be associated with an infection or with chemical irritants.

Key symptoms

• Pain in the tonsil and throat area.

• Difficulty in swallowing.

• Throat has a red colouration.

• Loss of voice or hoarse voice.

• Fever or cold may be present or about to start.

> DR: Throat cervical spine and neck area.
>
> AR: All toes, lymph system and adrenals.

Sore throats may be a sign of a more serious condition, and should be checked by a doctor.

CONJUNCTIVITIS AND BLEPHARITIS

Both these conditions may be caused by a physical or a chemical irritant and/or infection. Conjunctivitis is the inflammation of the conjunctiva, the mucous membrane that covers the eyeball. The edges of the eyelid become inflamed in blepharitis.

Key symptoms for conjunctivitis

• Discharge of water or pus from the eye.

• Eyes are red or pink.

• 'Gritty' feeling in the eye.

• Increased sensitivity to light.

• Soreness or swelling.

• The vision may be slightly blurred.

Key symptoms of blepharitis

• Painful, red, scaly eyelids.

• The eyelids often have a crust over them.

> DR: Eyes.
>
> AR: Neck, cervical spine, kidneys, adrenal glands and upper lymphatics.

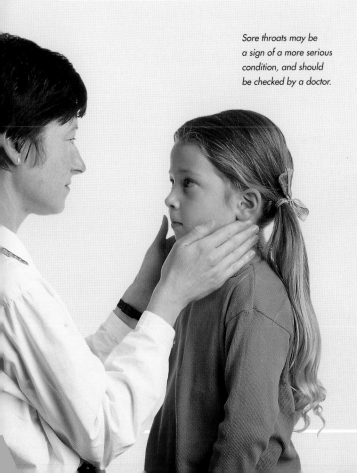

The skin on our hands is particularly exposed and so may be vulnerable to certain skin conditions.

Skin and Hair Problems

The skin is the largest organ in the body, so it's not surprising that even minor skin disorders can cause a lot of suffering.

ECZEMA

Skin that is inflamed and itchy. This may be associated with allergies, nervous stress or chemical or metal irritants. Eczema can affect all parts of the body or it can be localized, depending on the cause. It is often a hereditary condition.

Key symptoms

• Itchy, red, inflamed patches, which may bleed.

• Flaking skin which sometimes cracks forming raw patches, followed by a crust.

DR: Reflex area corresponding to the body part covered by the affected area of skin.
AR: Pituitary, adrenal glands, thyroid, kidney, lymphatics, solar plexus and the intestines.

PSORIASIS

This is a common skin disorder in which the skin produces too many skin cells. It is commonly found over the knees, elbows, trunk and scalp. It may be caused by stress, and/or a nervous, introverted personality. Psoriasis is often an inherited condition. Sometimes cutting out red meat from the diet acts as a remedy.

Key symptoms

• Patches of red, scaly skin.

• This condition can be quite unsightly and embarrassing for the sufferers.

• This condition has periods of remission and recurrence.

DR: Reflex area corresponding to the body part covered by the affected area of skin.
AR: Thyroid, adrenals, kidneys, liver, diaphragm, solar plexus, intestine and the lymphatics.

There is a lot of pressure on us to always look our best, and among other things this can result in excessive hair-washing, which will irritate the scalp.

ACNE

This condition is especially common among teenagers. It occurs where the sebaceous glands in the skin become infected, usually on the face, back or chest.

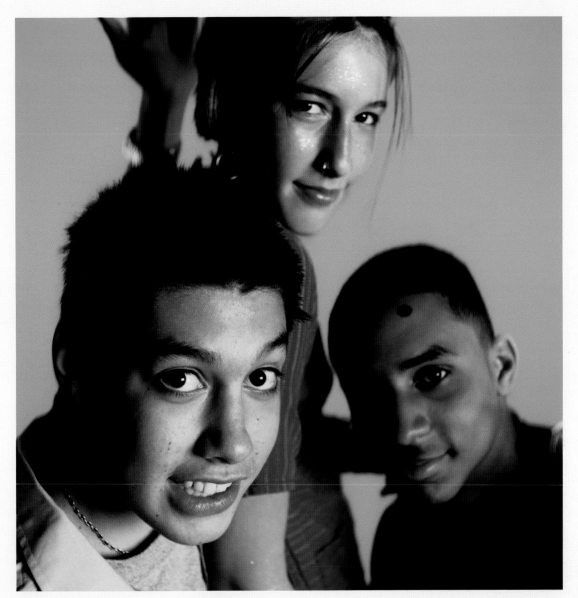

Key symptoms

• Area covered in red, angry-looking spots, which may contain pus.

• Very oily skin.

• Scarring in severe cases.

DR: Reflex area corresponding to the body part covered by the affected area of skin.

AR: All the glands, kidneys, liver and lymphatics.

Allergies

Allergies occur when our immune systems respond to organic triggers, or 'allergens'. These provoke an extreme immune response in some people, and the symptoms (streaming eyes, sweating, rashes) are the result of the body's attempts to rid itself of the allergen.

HAY FEVER

This is when the mucous membranes of the respiratory system become inflamed because of allergies to dust pollen or other air-borne substances.

Key symptoms

• Runny nose and sneezing.

• Eyes may be sore and red, and can be either dry or watery.

• Itchy eyes and respiratory tract.

• Wheezing may occur in severe cases.

DR: Eyes, sinuses, the head and the respiratory system.
AR: Adrenal glands, spleen, upper lymphatics and large intestine.

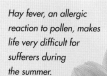

Hay fever, an allergic reaction to pollen, makes life very difficult for sufferers during the summer.

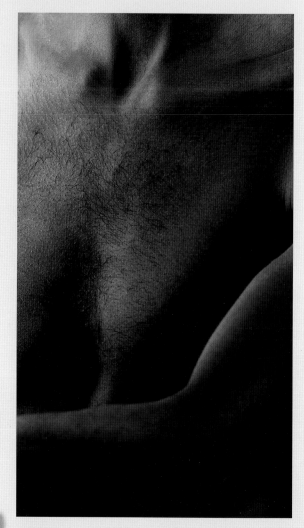

The immune system affects the whole body. The best way to avoid ill-health is to bolster the immune system with a proper diet and regular exercise.

URTICARIA,

HIVES OR NETTLE RASH

This is an allergic reaction of the skin to allergens. These allergens may be food (milk, eggs, shellfish and nuts are a few of the more common ones), environmental (cold, sunlight or heat), stress, anxiety, or bites or stings.

BEES

Key symptoms

• White or yellow itchy swellings surrounded by red inflamed skin.

• The swellings may join together to form a rash.

The skin may have an allergic reaction to a wide variety of allergens, from bee stings to sunlight.

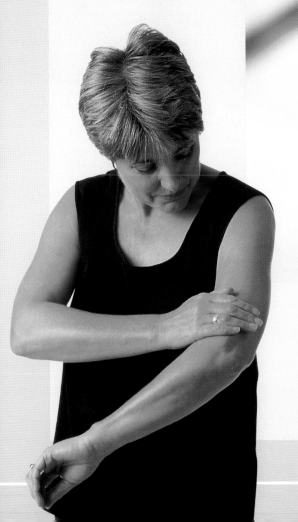

DR: Reflex area corresponding to the body part covered by the affected area of skin.

AR: Thyroid, adrenals, kidneys, liver, diaphragm, solar plexus, intestine and lymphatics.

Nervous Disorders

Many nervous disorders have mental rather than physical causes, and so allopathic medicine may not always be very helpful. Reflexology is a good way to encourage people to relax, and so it is a useful tool in these conditions.

INSOMNIA

This is a common complaint, with one third of the adult population suffering at some stage of their life. Insomnia is a condition in which the person cannot get to sleep, or has difficulties in staying asleep. Insomnia is often caused by worry or stress.

Key symptoms

• Difficulty in getting to sleep, or difficulty in staying asleep.
• Poor quality of sleep.

DR: Brain.
AR: All toes, all glands, solar plexus, and diaphragm.

Most of us suffer from the occasional bad night's sleep, but for some people insomnia can become a debilitating condition.

ANXIETY AND DEPRESSION

These two conditions are often associated with each other. Everyone is anxious at some time, but excessive feelings of worry and doom can lead to serious physical and psychological problems, and so should be treated.

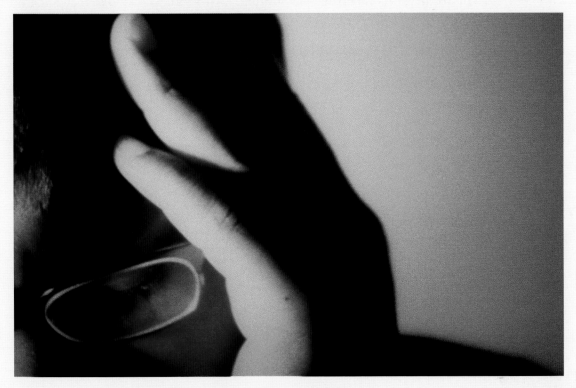

A surprisingly large proportion of the adult population will be affected by depression at some time in their lives.

Key symptoms

There are many physical signs linked to these conditions. Any combination of the following symptoms may be present.

- Being unable to relax.
- Headaches, palpitations, a rapid pulse, tightness in the chest, high blood pressure.
- Sleeplessness.
- Loss of appetite, nausea, diarrhoea.
- Light-headedness.

DR: Pituitary and head.
AR: All toes, all glands, solar plexus, diaphragm and intestines.

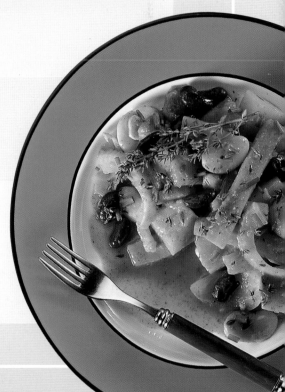

One of the warning signs of depression is a sudden loss of appetite. Be sure to consult your medical doctor if you think that you may be suffering.

Treating Yourself

If you are suffering from a serious disorder, or if you are new to reflexology, it is best to consult a qualified practitioner at first. However, you will soon pick up ways of treating yourself at home.

The hands are much better suited to self-treatment than the feet, as they are more accessible.

You can use reflexology to treat yourself. Giving yourself a hand treatment is not only easier, in terms of comfort, than the feet, but is also more convenient, as it can be carried out in any place, at any time. The desired effects are the same. Like the feet, the hands reflect all the body. They are a different shape, but once the basic layout has been learnt the location of the reflexes is quite straightforward. The main difference between the hands and the feet is that the areas are more condensed in the hands. The hands are also usually exposed to the elements, and so are not as sensitive as the feet. Generally this will mean that more treatments will be required for hand reflexology than for foot reflexology.

You cannot harm yourself by carrying out a self-treatment. Care should, however, be taken not to over-stimulate one area, as this may lead to your energies being unbalanced.

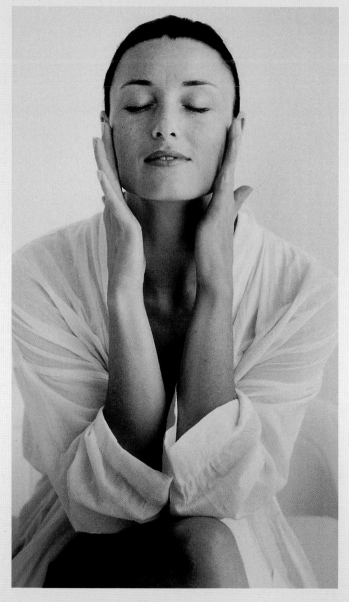

Self-treatment with reflexology will have a relaxing and revitalising effect.

THE ANATOMY OF THE HAND

The foot and hand have similar basic structures. The hand, which does not have to bear the full weight of the body, is more delicate, with long, mobile fingers.

The thumb is made up of two phalanges and the four fingers each have three phalanges.

At the base of each of the phalanges is a metacarpal bone. The five metacarpal bones form the palm of the hand. The eight carpal bones are made up of the trapezium, which is under the thumb metacarpal; the trapezoid, under the index finger metacarpal; the capitate, under the middle finger metacarpal; and the hamate, under the fourth and fifth metacarpals. The scaphoid lunate, triquetral and pisiform are found in the wrist.

The mobility of the carpal bones, along with the associated muscles, tendons and ligaments, which also keep the bones in place, make the hand a very flexible and precise tool.

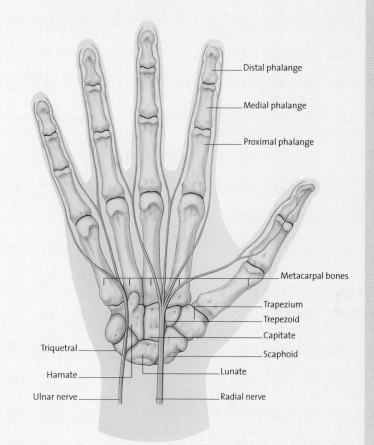

Distal phalange

Medial phalange

Proximal phalange

Metacarpal bones

Trapezium

Trepezoid

Capitate

Scaphoid

Triquetral

Lunate

Hamate

Ulnar nerve

Radial nerve

The human hand, with its opposable thumb, is one of the most delicate and versatile tools in nature, and can perform a great variety of tasks with ease.

Reflex maps of the Hands and their Relationship to Body Parts

The hand, like the foot, is divided into five longitudinal zones. Also like the foot, the left hand represents the left-hand side of the body, and the left brain. The right hand represents the right-hand side of the body, and the right brain. The reflexes in the hand on the whole occupy similar positions to those on the foot.

THE HAND

The hand, because of its shape and size, can be divided into seven sections, as follows.

• The head and neck. This is represented by the fingers.

• The thoracic and upper abdominal area. This area includes the shoulder, lungs, diaphragm, most of the stomach and liver, and part of the kidneys. The waistline on the hand is harder to identify than on the foot. It is found at the base of the metacarpals.

• The lower abdominal area and pelvic areas are found over the carpal bones.

• The reproductive area is represented by parts of the wrist.

• The spine is represented by the outside edge of the thumb, running down until it meets the wrist, where it goes across the wrist.

• The limb reflexes are found on the little finger side of the hand.

• The breast and lymphatics reflexes are found on the back of the hand.

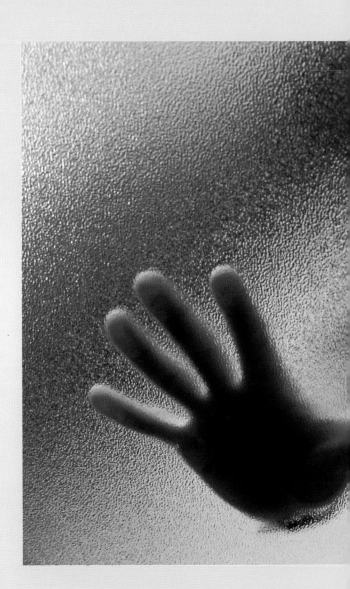

When you are feeling stressed or out of kilter, give yourself a hand reflexology treatment. You will feel better for it.

BASIC TECHNIQUE

The technique for giving yourself a treatment on the hands is the same as that for giving a foot reflexology treatment. As the hands are smaller, it usually takes less time, and greater precision is required, but it should be just as enjoyable. Enjoy giving treatments to yourself and others. It will be a marvellous hour of health-giving relaxation for both you and your clients.

Relax your hands before starting on a self-treatment.

The **Head**

The most common ailment related to this area is, of course, headaches. If you suffer from headaches, try to keep your head and neck mobile throughout the day; localized stiffening of the muscles in the neck and at the base of the skull leads to classic tension headaches.

The following reflexes in the head are found in both the hands.

• The thumb represents one half of the head. The top of the head reflex is found at the top of the thumb, next to the nail.

• The pituitary gland reflex is found roughly in the middle of the fleshy part of the thumb.

• The brain reflex is found towards the top part of the thumb.

• The face reflex is found on the front of the thumb, under the nail.

• The side of the head and side of the brain reflexes are found on the side of the thumb, which is next to the index finger.

• The neck reflex and throat reflex are found in the second joint of the thumb.

• The four fingers represent the sinus reflexes on the palm side, and the teeth reflexes are on the back of the hands.

• The eye reflex is found at the base of the index and middle fingers.

• The ear reflex is found at the base of the fourth and little fingers.

• The Eustachian tube reflex is found in the webbing and fleshy part of the skin between the middle and fourth finger, both on the front and back of the hands.

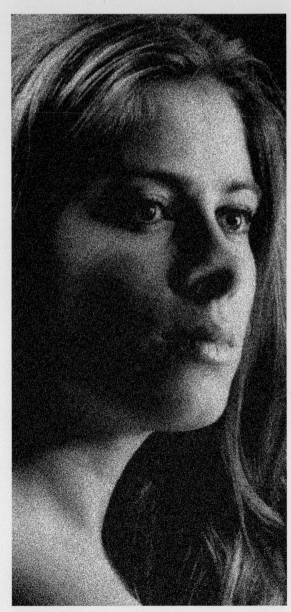

In common with mice and giraffes, humans have seven neck vertebrae, which must support the whole weight of the head.

HEAD REFLEX POINTS

LEFT HAND

The Eustachian tube reflex is found in the webbing and fleshy part of the skin between the middle and fourth fingers.

Eustachian tube

RIGHT HAND

Teeth and gums

Brain

Face

The brain reflex is found towards the top point of the thumb.

Sinuses

LEFT HAND

Eyes

Brain

Pituitary

Eustachian tube

Ears

Neck and thyroid

The side of the head and side of the brain reflexes are found on the side of the thumb next to the index finger.

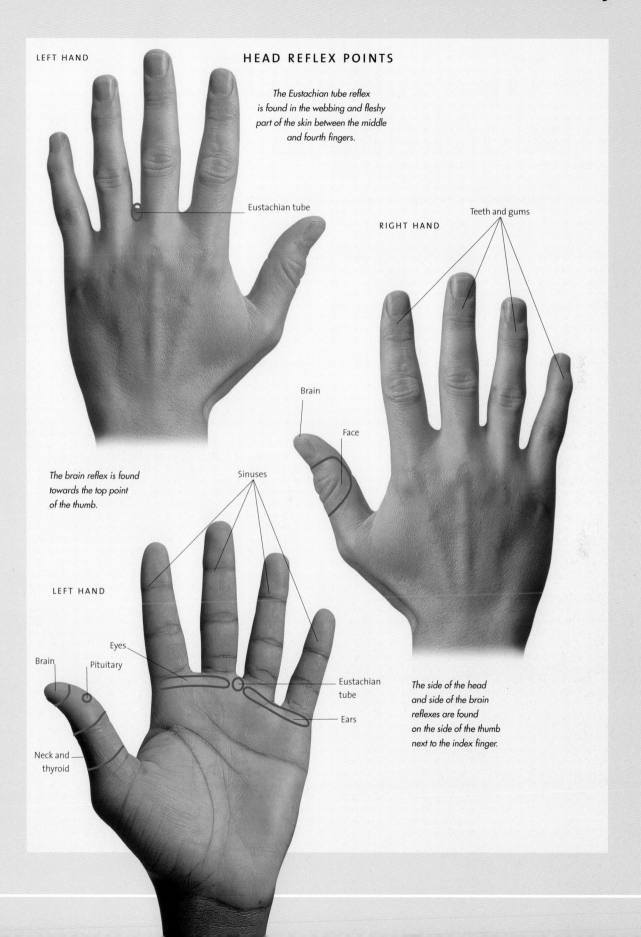

The **Thoracic** and **Upper Abdominal** Area

This area of the hand contains several vital reflexes, including the heart, lungs, thyroid and thymus glands, diaphragm, solar plexus, liver, stomach, pancreas, spleen and kidney. Maintaining good energy flow through this area is essential for good health.

• The shoulder reflex is found at the base of the little finger, both on the palm and the back of both of the hands.

• The lung reflex is found under the fingers on both the palm side and on the back of both of the hands. The lung reflex crosses all 4 zones.

• The diaphragm reflex is found where the phalanges meet the metacarpals, across the 5 zones on both of the hands.

• The heart reflex, as in the foot, is an exception to the rule. It is found in the left hand in zones 2 to 3, above the diaphragm reflex and near the lung reflex.

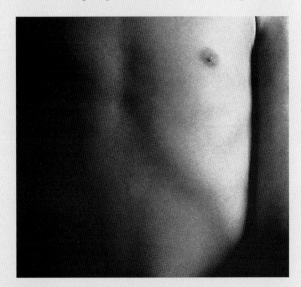

Many major organs are housed in the upper part of the abdomen, so this is a vital area to work on.

• The thyroid reflex is found at the base of the thumb, below the neck reflex. It stretches across the whole of the palm side of the thumb (zone 1), and the parathyroid reflex is found in that area of the thumb that is close to the index finger, below the neck reflex. As in the foot, there is an upper and lower parathyroid reflex.

• The solar plexus reflex is found at the same level as the diaphragm reflex in zone 3 of the palm side of both hands.

• The liver reflex is found in the palm of the right hand. As in the foot, it is found between the diaphragm and waistline, filling up most of this area, and the area between zones 3 to 5.

• The gallbladder reflex is found in zone 4 in roughly the middle of the liver reflex.

• The stomach reflex is found on both palms. On the left palm it occupies zones 1 to 4; on the right hand it occupies zone 1. The reflex lies between the diaphragm reflex and the waistline.

• The pancreas reflex is found in a similar area to the stomach reflex.

• The spleen reflex is found on the palm of the left hand between zones 4 and 5.

• The kidney reflexes are found on the palms of both hands at about waistline level in zones 2 to 3.

• The adrenal reflexes are found on the palms of both hands just above and towards the outside of the kidney reflex in zone 2.

THORACIC AND ABDOMINAL
REFLEX POINTS

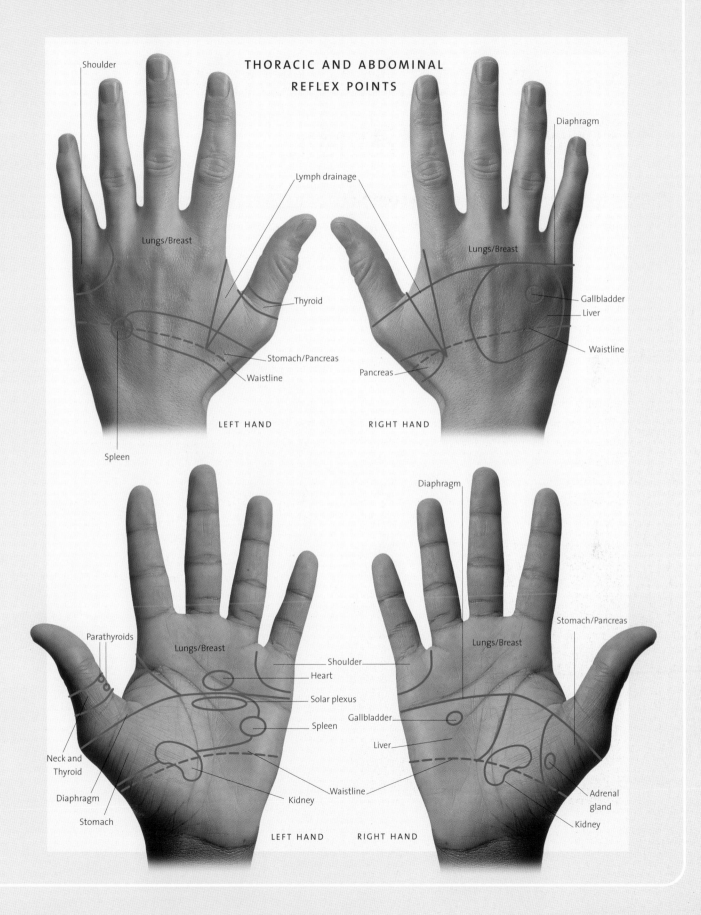

Shoulder

Lymph drainage

Lungs/Breast

Thyroid

Stomach/Pancreas

Waistline

Spleen

LEFT HAND

Diaphragm

Lungs/Breast

Gallbladder

Liver

Waistline

Pancreas

RIGHT HAND

Parathyroids

Lungs/Breast

Shoulder

Heart

Solar plexus

Spleen

Neck and Thyroid

Diaphragm

Stomach

Waistline

Kidney

LEFT HAND

Diaphragm

Stomach/Pancreas

Lungs/Breast

Gallbladder

Liver

Adrenal gland

Kidney

RIGHT HAND

The **Lower Abdominal** and **Pelvic** Areas

A sluggish digestion and ailments of the genito-urinary system will respond well to treatments with reflexology. How to find the necessary reflex points is outlined here.

• The small intestine reflex is found in the palms of both hands, in between the waistline and just above the wrist from zones 1 to 4.

• The ileo-caecal valve reflex is found on the right palm, in between zones 4 and 5, away from the wrist.

• The appendix reflex, as in the feet, is at the same location as the ileo-caecal valve reflex.

• The large intestine reflex is found on the palms of both hands. The form it takes is the same as in the feet. It starts on the right palm at the ileo-caecal valve reflex and goes up, representing the ascending colon reflex; it turns at a right angle just below the waistline to become the transverse colon reflex, which goes across the palm of the hand; and it extends across into the left hand, and across all the five zones. At the spleen reflex, between zones 4 and 5, it takes another right-angle bend down into the descending colon reflex. A short distance above the wrist, another right-angle turn is made into the sigmoid reflex, which extends across the palm above the wrist and ends in the rectum reflex.

• The ureter reflex is found in the palms of both hands, linking the kidney reflex to the bladder reflex.

• The bladder reflex is found on the outer side of zone 1, just above the rectum reflex.

• The sciatic reflex is found in the palms of both hands, close to the wrist and extending across all five zones, along the wrist line.

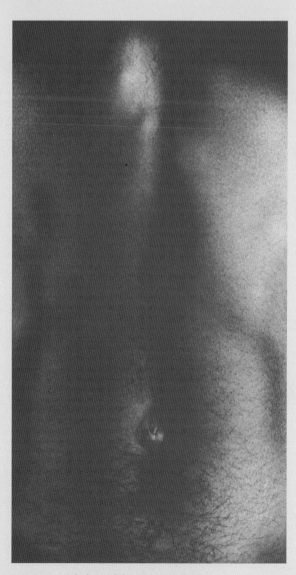

The lower abdomen contains the digestive system and the genito-urinary system, and is important to all-round good health.

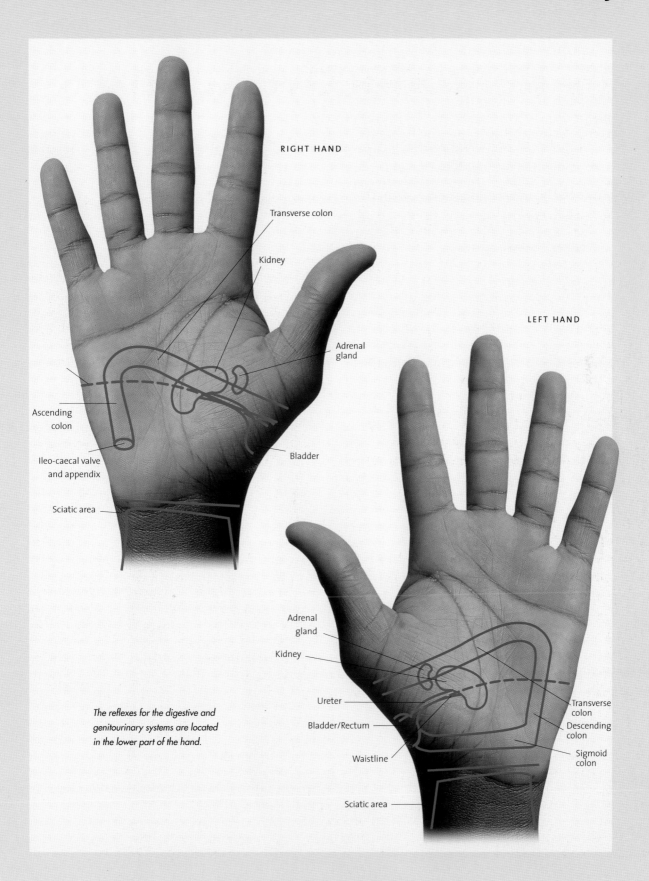

RIGHT HAND

Transverse colon

Kidney

LEFT HAND

Adrenal gland

Ascending colon

Bladder

Ileo-caecal valve and appendix

Sciatic area

Adrenal gland

Kidney

The reflexes for the digestive and genitourinary systems are located in the lower part of the hand.

Ureter

Bladder/Rectum

Transverse colon

Descending colon

Waistline

Sigmoid colon

Sciatic area

The **Reproductive Reflexes**

The reproductive reflexes have a similar arrangement in the hands to those in the feet. The reflexes are present on both the palms and the tops of both of the hands just above the wrist.

- The ovary/testes reflexes are found zone 5.
- The uterus/prostate reflexes are found in zone 1.
- The Fallopian tube and seminal vesicle/vas deferens reflex is found across the top of the hand, linking the ovary/testes reflexes with the uterus/prostate reflexes.

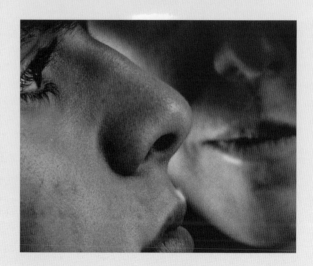

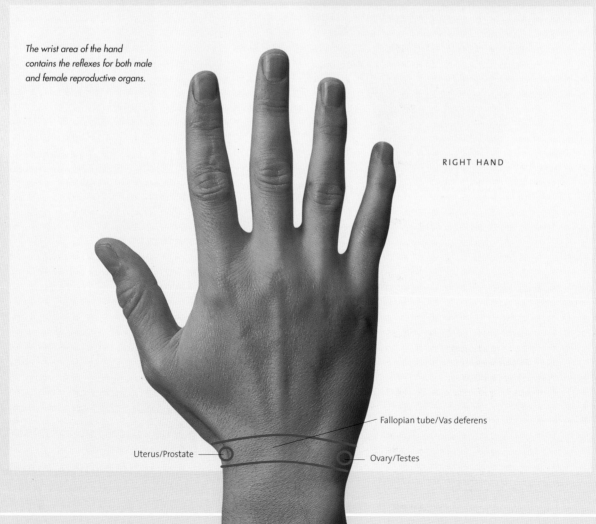

The wrist area of the hand contains the reflexes for both male and female reproductive organs.

RIGHT HAND

Fallopian tube/Vas deferens

Uterus/Prostate

Ovary/Testes

The **Spine**

The spine: one of the most crucial parts of the body, and the source of some common complaints.

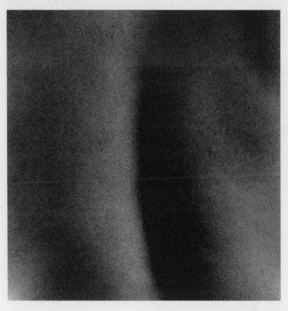

When treating the spine reflex on the hand, be especially sensitive to any sensations that are felt by you or the client, as these will tell you which areas need to be reworked.

• The spine reflex is represented by the outside of the thumb, running down and then across that fleshy part of the hand between the palm and wrist, stopping at the other side of the wrist. The various parts of the spine are again distinguishable from one another.

SPINE REFLEX POINTS

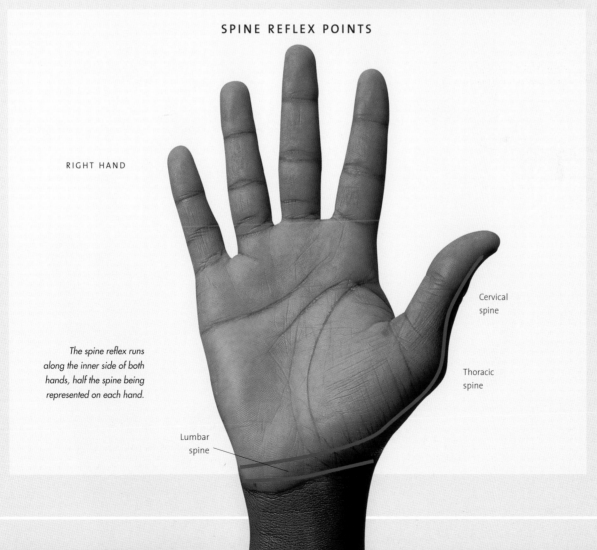

RIGHT HAND

The spine reflex runs along the inner side of both hands, half the spine being represented on each hand.

Cervical spine

Thoracic spine

Lumbar spine

The **Limb Reflexes**

As with the feet, the reflex points that refer to bodily extremities are on the outsides of the hands.

If you suffer from varicose veins or pins and needles in your legs, make a conscious effort not to cross your legs at the knee. Try to cross them at the ankles instead.

• The arm reflex is found on the outer side of zone 5, under the shoulder reflex on the back of both hands.
• The hip and knee reflexes are found on the back of both hands on the outer side of zone 5.

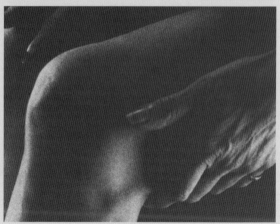

LIMB REFLEX POINTS

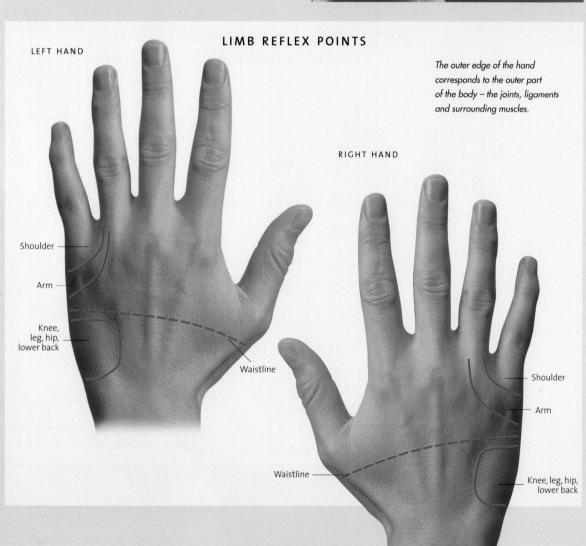

LEFT HAND

The outer edge of the hand corresponds to the outer part of the body – the joints, ligaments and surrounding muscles.

RIGHT HAND

Shoulder

Arm

Knee, leg, hip, lower back

Waistline

Shoulder

Arm

Waistline

Knee, leg, hip, lower back

Lymphatics and Breast Area

As previously discussed, the lymphatic system – which transports the lymph around the body – has profound effects on our overall well-being, so it is worth paying attention to this area when you treat yourself or other people.

• The breast reflex is found on the back of both hands, above the waistline, across zones 2 to 4.
• The upper lymph nodes reflexes are found in the webbing between the fingers.
• The lymph nodes of the groin reflex is found across zones 1 to 5, just above the wrist.

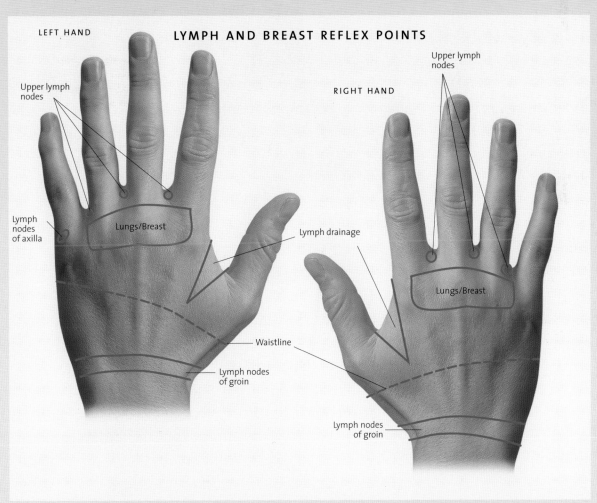

LEFT HAND   **LYMPH AND BREAST REFLEX POINTS**

Upper lymph nodes

RIGHT HAND

Upper lymph nodes

Upper lymph nodes

Lymph nodes of axilla

Lungs/Breast

Lymph drainage

Lungs/Breast

Waistline

Lymph nodes of groin

Lymph nodes of groin

Glossary

ABDOMINAL AREA The area of the body that starts at the diaphragm and extends under the lungs to the genitals.

CARDIOVASCULAR Concerning the heart and/or the circulatory system.

CASE HISTORY This is where the therapist asks the client personal details, such as their medical history and occupation.

CONGESTION In reflexology this means an area of the body where there is not a free flow of energy.

HEALING CRISIS This is the process by which a patient gets rid of toxic substances, sometimes causing them to feel unwell.

HOLISTIC Taken from the Greek word *Holas*, which means 'whole'. In reflexology it means that the person is treated as a whole, on a physical, mental and spiritual level.

ORGAN A multicellular part of an animal, which forms a structural unit (e.g. the liver).

REFLEX An area found on the feet and hands that corresponds to a gland, an organ or a part of the body.

THORACIC AREA The area containing the heart and lungs. It is clearly marked off from the abdomen by the diaphragm.

TOXINS These are essentially poisons, which may be created by the body, ingested in the food we eat or drink or may enter the body by other means.

VITAL FORCE This is the same thing as the life force. It is the energy within us. Without it we cannot live.

WAISTLINE An imaginary line running horizontally across the foot and hand. On the foot it runs from the cuboid notch across to the other side of the foot.

ZONE In reflexology, any one of ten longitudinal sections through the body. Each zone contains one finger (or thumb) and one toe.

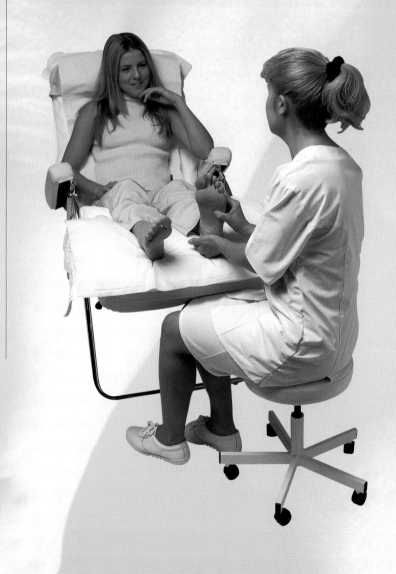

Useful Addresses

Association of Reflexologists
27 Old Gloucester Street
London
WC1N 3XX
Tel: 0870 5673320

Bayly School of Reflexology
Monks Orchard
Whitbourne
Worcs
WR6 5RB
Tel/Fax: 01886 821207
email: bayly@britreflex.co.uk
www.britreflex.co.uk

BCMA (British Complementary
Medicine Association)
33 Imperial Square
Cheltenham
Glos
GL0 1QZ
Tel: 0845 3455977
email: info@bcma.co.uk
www.bcma.co.uk

British School of Reflexology and Holistic
Association of Reflexologists
(BSR Sales Limited)
92 Sheering Road
Old Harlow
Essex
CM17 0JW
Tel: 01279 429066
Fax: 01279 445234
www.footreflexology.com

Chrysalis School of Reflexology
14 Central Avenue
Cooktown
County Tyrone
Northern Ireland
BT80 8AJ
Tel: 028 86763664

Colour and Reflexology
(contact: Pauline Wills)
9 Wyndale Avenue
Kingsbury
London
NW9 9PT
Tel/Fax: 020 82047672
email: pauline@oracleschoolstreet.co.uk

International Federation of Reflexologists
76–8 Edridge Road
Croydon
Surrey
CR0 1EF
Tel: 020 86679458
Fax: 020 86499291
www.reflexology-ifr.com

Irish Reflexologists' Institute
3 Blackglen Court
Lambs Cross
Sandyford
Dublin
Republic of Ireland

Scottish Institute of Reflexology
(contact: Margaret Whittington)
'Taymount'
Hill Crescent
Wormit
Fife
BD6 8PQ
Tel: 01382 541372

Index

aches and pains 70–1
Achilles tendon stretch 45
acupuncture 19
allergies 76–7
anatomy 12–19, 24–5, 81
ankle rotation 45
arteriosclerosis 10, 62

Bayly, Doreen 7
benefits 11
bladder 21, 31, 36, 67, 88
breasts 25, 37, 82, 93

case histories 38–9
caterpillar walk (CW) 42,
    47–55
circulatory system 9–10, 13,
    56, 62–3
creative cycle 20

destructive cycle 21
digestive system 16, 64–7
diseases 58–79

ears 17, 26, 72, 84
earth 20–1
elements 20–1
endocrine system 15, 29
eyes 17, 26, 57, 73, 84

fire 20–1
Fitzgerald, William 7
foot wobbling 45
fungal infections 41, 57

gallbladder 21, 65, 86

head 24, 26–7, 82, 84–5
healing crisis 56–7
heart 21, 28, 57, 62–3, 86
homeostasis 9

icons 21
Ingham, Eunice 7, 10

kidneys 21, 25, 86

large intestine 21, 30–1, 88
life force 8–9
limbs 25, 36, 92
liver 21, 67, 82, 86
lower abdomen 25, 30–1,
    82, 88–9
lymphatic system 14, 25, 37,
    82, 93

maps 22–3, 82–3
meridians 19
metal 20–1
metatarsal kneading 44
mouth 72–3
muscular system 12

neck 24, 26, 82, 84
nervous system 9, 11, 13, 22,
    78–9
nose 18

pelvis 25, 32, 36, 82, 88–9
pericardium 21
precautions 41, 57
preparations 40

reactions 56–7, 59
reproductive system 16, 25,
    33, 36, 68–9, 82, 90
respiratory system 14, 60–1

self-treatments 80–1
sensory system 17
sinuses 26, 61, 84
skeletal system 12
skin 17, 74–5
small intestine 21, 30, 88
spinal twist 45
spine 25, 34–5, 57, 82, 91
spleen 21, 29, 86, 88
stomach 21, 25, 29, 82, 86

talcum powder 42
techniques
    basic 40–3, 82
    main treatment 46–55
    relaxation 43–5
    self-treatment 80–1
thoracic area 24, 28–9, 82,
    86–7
throat 72–3, 84
thumb-rolling 44
toe rotation 44
tongue 18
toxins 9, 19, 56

upper abdomen 24, 28–9,
    82, 86–7
urinary system 15

varicose veins 41, 65
vital energy 8–9

waistline 24–5, 82
water 20–1
wood 20–1

zone therapy 7

Acknowledgements

Special thanks go to
Sarah Allaway for photography
co-ordination
Malika Hopkins and
Joëlle Peeters for help with
photography

*The publishers would like to thank
the following for the use of pictures:*
Image Bank 80
Images Colour Library 67,
69, 77, 82/83
Stockmarket 6
Stone Gettyone 1, 8, 10,
17, 18, 22, 24/25, 39, 56/57,
58, 63, 75, 79

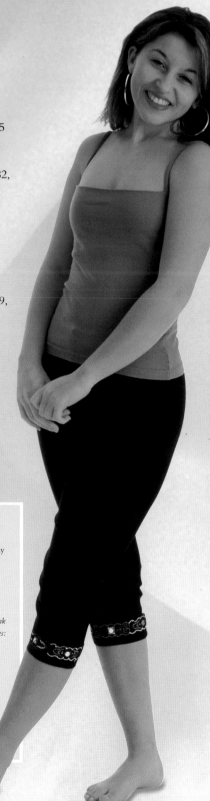